Introduction to Exam 2

Structure of Exam 2

Content outline 2

    Basic Sciences 2

    Equipment, Instrumentation, and Technology 2

    General Principles of Anesthesia 3

    Anesthesia for Surgical Procedures and Special Populations 3

Author Introduction 4

Study guide of NBCRNA SEE 5

NBCRNA Self-Evaluation Examination Practice Test 19

    Test Answer Key 72

Reward for the Readers 111

Introduction to Exam

The NBCRNA SEE exam is an important test for nurses who want to become nurse anesthetists. Nurse anesthetists are healthcare professionals who help doctors during surgeries and procedures by giving anesthesia, which helps patients not feel pain. This exam is administered by NBCRNA (National Board of Certification and Recertification for Nurse Anesthetists) to make sure nurses have the right knowledge and skills to work as nurse anesthetists safely. The exam is a computerized adaptive test designed to evaluate the strengths and weaknesses of both students and programs before the NCE. Passing the exam is a big achievement and shows that nurses are ready to work as nurse anesthetists. You will need to study hard and do well on the NBCRNA SEE exam if you want to become a nurse anesthetist.

Structure of Exam

The exam is presented on a computer screen, with questions displayed one at a time. Throughout the four-hour testing period, students must answer a total of 240 questions. It consists of multiple-choice questions and various alternative question formats like multiple correct responses, calculations, hotspots, and drag and drop. This format allows for a comprehensive assessment of students' knowledge and skills, ensuring they are well-prepared for certification as nurse anesthetists.

Content outline

There are four main domains of the NBCRNA SEE exam.

Basic Sciences

In this domain, you will dive into the building blocks of anesthesia practice. First up, anatomy and physiology—this covers understanding the body's structures and how they function. Then there is pathophysiology, which focuses on what goes wrong when diseases or conditions disrupt normal bodily processes. Pharmacology comes next, dealing with medications and how they interact with the body. Lastly, you will tackle applied chemistry, biochemistry, physics, and math. Here, you will explore how these sciences are used in anesthesia practice, such as understanding drug reactions, gas laws for breathing, and calculating medication doses.

Equipment, Instrumentation, and Technology

In this domain, you will explore the tools of the trade in anesthesia practice. First off, there are anesthetic delivery systems, which are the machines that help administer anesthesia gases or medications to patients. Then, you will learn about airway equipment—devices used to keep a patient's airway open during anesthesia. Monitoring devices come next, which help keep track of vital signs like heart rate and oxygen levels during surgery. Patient warming equipment is also covered, which helps maintain a patient's body temperature. Infusion devices, like rapid infusers, are important for delivering medications and fluids accurately and efficiently. Lastly, you will study imaging and imaging safety, understanding how certain medical imaging techniques can aid in anesthesia procedures and ensuring safety protocols are followed. Mastering these tools and technologies is crucial for providing safe and effective anesthesia care.

General Principles of Anesthesia

In this domain, you will cover a wide range of important topics essential for safe and effective anesthesia care. Firstly, ethical considerations and legal issues are discussed, ensuring that patient rights and professional responsibilities are upheld. Safety and wellness are emphasized to protect both patients and healthcare providers during procedures. Preoperative assessment and preparation of patients involve thorough evaluations to ensure they are ready for surgery. Fluid volume assessment and management are crucial for maintaining patient hydration and stability. Airway management is a key skill, ensuring patients can breathe properly during anesthesia. Techniques for administering local/regional anesthetics and managing complications are taught, along with methods for sedation and pain management. Other topics include enhanced recovery after surgery, hypotensive technique, infection control, and fire safety in the operating room. Understanding these principles is essential for providing high-quality anesthesia care and promoting positive patient outcomes.

Anesthesia for Surgical Procedures and Special Populations

In this domain, you will delve into the specifics of administering anesthesia during various surgical procedures and for patients with special needs. Firstly, you will learn about surgical and diagnostic anesthesia, which involves understanding how to provide anesthesia tailored to different types of surgeries while managing any complications that may arise during the procedure. This includes techniques for maintaining patient comfort and safety throughout the surgical process. Additionally, you will study anesthesia for special populations, like pediatric patients, elderly individuals, or those with specific medical conditions. This entails adapting anesthesia techniques and dosages to meet the unique needs and considerations of these patient groups, ensuring they receive optimal care and minimizing any risks associated with anesthesia administration. Mastering these skills is essential for providing safe and effective anesthesia to all patients undergoing surgical procedures.

Author Introduction

As your reliable guide and author through the NBCRNA SEE Exam, I bring a wealth of experience and expertise in anesthesia practice. My goal is to assist you in navigating the difficulties of this exam with confidence, simplifying complex concepts along the way. I am dedicated to equipping you with the necessary skills to excel in anesthesia practice and thrive in your professional activities beyond simply passing the exam. I am committed to providing comprehensive support throughout your preparation process with a focus on personalized guidance tailored to your needs. I am here to offer practical insights and assistance at every stage of your journey as an experienced instructor in anesthesia practice. Together, we will ensure you are fully prepared to tackle the NBCRNA SEE Exam and embark on a successful career path in anesthesia practice with confidence and competence.

As a single author, some mistakes are still possible if you find any mistake, please send me an email by scanning the QR code so I can update this and give you a better reward:

Study guide of NBCRNA SEE

Introduction

Here is the study guide for the NBCRNA SEE (National Board of Certification and Recertification for Nurse Anesthetists Self-Evaluation Examination). This guide is designed to provide aspiring nurse anesthetists with the fundamental knowledge and resources required to succeed in their certification process. Within healthcare, the field of nurse anesthesia plays an important part in providing secure and effective anesthesia care. Therefore, passing the NBCRNA SEE exam is a crucial milestone on the way to becoming a Certified Registered Nurse Anesthetist (CRNA). This guide offers invaluable information and support for your professional growth in nurse anesthesia, whether you are a practicing nurse seeking recertification or a nursing student preparing for certification.

Overview of Nurse Anesthesia Profession

Nurse anesthesia has a rich history that dates back to the Civil War era when nurses first began administering anesthesia to wounded soldiers. Over the years, the profession has evolved significantly, with nurse anesthetists now recognized as highly skilled advanced practice registered nurses (APRNs). Certified Registered Nurse Anesthetists (CRNAs) play a crucial role in the healthcare system by providing anesthesia care to patients undergoing surgical procedures. Their scope of practice encompasses not only the administration of anesthesia but also the monitoring of patients throughout surgery and the provision of post-anesthesia care. Anesthesia is essential in modern healthcare as it ensures patient comfort and safety during medical procedures. CRNAs work closely with other healthcare professionals, including surgeons, anesthesiologists, and nurses, in the perioperative setting to ensure optimal patient outcomes. Such collaboration is vital for coordinating care and addressing any potential complications that may arise during surgery.

Content outline

There are four main domains of the SEE exam which are as follows:

1. Basic Sciences

This domain covers fundamental scientific principles essential for understanding anesthesia practice. Topics covered include physics, anatomy, physiology, pharmacology, and biochemistry, which offer a strong foundation for safe and effective anesthesia administration. Subcategories of basic sciences include:

Anatomy and Physiology

The subdomain of Basic Sciences comprises the cardiovascular, respiratory, central nervous system, musculoskeletal, endocrine, hepatic and renal, hematologic, gastrointestinal, and immune systems. Understanding the structure and function of these systems is essential for CRNAs to assess, monitor, and manage patients' physiological responses during anesthesia.

Pathophysiology

Cardiovascular:

Ischemic heart disease: Refers to conditions such as angina and myocardial infarction (heart attack) caused by reduced blood flow to the heart.

Valvular heart disease: Involves abnormalities of the heart valves, which can affect blood flow within the heart.

Congenital heart defects: Structural abnormalities of the heart present at birth, ranging from minor defects to complex malformations.

Cardiac conduction and rhythm abnormalities: Disruptions in the heart's electrical conduction system cause irregular heartbeats.

Cardiovascular and peripheral vascular abnormalities: Various conditions, including arterial and venous diseases, affect blood vessels.

Infectious diseases: Cardiovascular infections, such as endocarditis, pericarditis, or those affecting blood vessels, pose significant health risks.

Pericardial diseases: These disorders involve the pericardium, the protective sac around the heart.

Cardiomyopathy and heart failure: Heart muscle diseases impair the heart's pumping ability, which leads to heart failure.

Respiratory:

Obstructive diseases: Respiratory conditions marked by airflow obstruction, including asthma, COPD, and bronchiectasis.

Restrictive diseases: Disorders diminishing lung volume and impeding lung expansion, such as interstitial lung diseases or chest wall deformities.

Infectious diseases: Respiratory tract infections like pneumonia, bronchitis, or tuberculosis.

Pulmonary vascular abnormalities: Disorders impacting blood vessels within the lungs, such as pulmonary embolism or pulmonary hypertension.

Altered airway anatomy: Variations or irregularities in airway structure potentially affecting anesthesia management.

Central nervous system:

Neurodegenerative diseases: Progressive nervous system disorders like Alzheimer's or Parkinson's.

Myelin diseases: Conditions causing damage to the myelin sheath, as seen in multiple sclerosis.

Cerebrovascular diseases: Disorders impacting blood flow to the brain, such as strokes or transient ischemic attacks.

Neuropathies: Nerve damage leading to sensory, motor, or autonomic disturbances.

Psychiatric disorders: Mental health conditions, including depression, anxiety, or schizophrenia.

Spinal cord disorders: Conditions affecting the spinal cord, such as injury or tumors.

Intracranial tumors: Abnormal growths within or around the brain.

Congenital abnormalities: Birth defects affecting brain or spinal cord structure or function.

Seizure disorders: Conditions marked by recurrent seizures or convulsions.

Intracranial hypertension: Increased pressure within the skull stemming from various causes.

Musculoskeletal:

Myopathies/metabolic abnormalities: Disorders impacting muscle function and metabolism comprise conditions like malignant hyperthermia.

Neuromuscular diseases: Conditions affecting nerves and muscles, such as myasthenia gravis or muscular dystrophy.

Skeletal diseases: Disorders involving bones, including osteoporosis, osteoarthritis, or fractures.

Musculoskeletal disorders: Genetic and acquired conditions may have an impact on the musculoskeletal system, potentially influencing positioning and mobility during surgery.

Endocrine:

Thyroid and parathyroid disorders: Dysfunction of the thyroid or parathyroid glands leads to hormonal imbalances.

Pituitary disorders: Abnormalities of the pituitary gland, which regulates various hormonal functions in the body.

Adrenal disorders: Dysfunction of the adrenal glands, resulting in hormonal imbalances like Addison's disease or Cushing's syndrome.

Pancreatic disorders (endocrine disorders): Conditions affecting the endocrine function of the pancreas, comprising diabetes mellitus and pancreatic endocrine tumors.

Other endocrine disorders include disorders that affect glands such as the thymus or hypothalamus and metabolic-related conditions like metabolic syndrome.

Hepatic:

Infectious diseases: Hepatitis or other infections affecting the liver.

Biliary tract and bilirubin disorders: Biliary tract and bilirubin disorders involve the bile ducts or metabolism of bilirubin.

Cirrhotic disorders: Chronic liver diseases leading to liver scarring and dysfunction.

Hepatovascular abnormalities: Conditions affecting blood flow within the liver, such as portal hypertension or hepatic artery thrombosis.

Renal:

Intrinsic kidney disorders: Diseases affecting the structure and function of the kidneys, including glomerulonephritis or polycystic kidney disease.

Acute kidney injury: Sudden loss of kidney function, often due to factors like dehydration, toxins, or reduced blood flow.

Chronic kidney disease: Progressive decline in kidney function over time, usually caused by conditions like diabetes or hypertension.

Hematologic:

Anemia: Conditions characterized by reduced red blood cell count or hemoglobin levels, such as iron deficiency anemia or sickle cell anemia.

Hemoglobin disorders: Abnormalities in the structure or function of hemoglobin, including thalassemia or hemoglobinopathies.

Coagulation disorders: Abnormalities in the blood clotting process that lead to bleeding disorders such as hemophilia or disseminated intravascular coagulation (DIC).

Gastrointestinal:

a. Esophageal disorders: Conditions affecting the tube connecting the throat to the stomach, like acid reflux or swallowing difficulties.

b. Gastric disorders: Problems with the stomach, such as ulcers, inflammation, or cancer.

c. Pancreatic disorders (exocrine disorders): Issues with the pancreas, like inflammation (pancreatitis) or cysts.

d. Intestinal disorders: Conditions affecting the intestines, including inflammation (Crohn's disease), infections, or blockages.

e. Tumors/secreting lesions: Abnormal growths or tissue changes in the gastrointestinal tract.

f. Malabsorption disorders: Conditions obstructing the absorption of nutrients from food, such as celiac disease or lactose intolerance.

Immune:

a. Infectious disorders (e.g., HIV, AIDS): Diseases caused by viruses or bacteria, such as HIV/AIDS.

b. Hypersensitivity disorders (Type I-IV): Allergic or immune reactions, ranging from hay fever to contact dermatitis.

c. Autoimmune diseases: Conditions where the immune system attacks the body's tissues, like rheumatoid arthritis or lupus.

Other conditions:

a. Cancer: Abnormal growths that can occur anywhere in the body.

b. Burns (inhalational, cutaneous): Injuries caused by heat, chemicals, or radiation.

c. Trauma: Physical injuries from accidents, falls, or violence.

d. Substance use disorder: Addiction to substances like alcohol, nicotine, or drugs.

e. Sepsis: A severe reaction to infection, leading to organ failure.

Pharmacology

Pharmacology encompasses different drug classes and their mechanisms of action, which are essential for anesthesia practice. General principles comprise pharmacodynamics, the study of how drugs affect the body, and pharmacokinetics, which examines drug absorption, distribution, metabolism, and excretion. Additionally, pharmacology-related mathematics are crucial for dosage calculations and drug administration. Inhalation anesthetics, intravenous anesthetics, and their antagonists are important in anesthesia induction and maintenance. These include barbiturates, sedatives/hypnotics like propofol and ketamine, benzodiazepines, opioids, and neuromuscular blockers. Local anesthetics offer regional anesthesia, while lipid emulsion helps treat local anesthetic toxicity. Adjuncts for regional anesthesia, such as anticholinergic and cholinergic agonists, improve block effectiveness. Other medication categories involve cardiovascular drugs, bronchodilators, psychopharmacologic agents, prostaglandins, insulin, diuretics, anticoagulants, antimicrobials, antiepileptics, lipid-lowering agents, and herbal remedies. To manage various clinical scenarios, knowledge of minerals, electrolytes, and drugs like dantrolene and steroids is essential. CRNAs providing optimal patient care emphasize the importance of pharmacological knowledge for safe and effective anesthesia management, ensuring understanding of these medications.

Applied chemistry, biochemistry, physics, and mathematics

Applied chemistry, biochemistry, physics, and mathematics form a foundational component of the NBCRNA SEE exam, providing CRNAs with essential knowledge for anesthesia practice. In chemistry and biochemistry, understanding aqueous solutions, acids, bases, salts, chemical reactions, metabolism, cellular mechanisms of action, and drug-receptor interactions is crucial for comprehending drug actions and interactions within the body. Physics principles encompass units of measurement, gas laws, solubility, pressure, fluid flow, electricity, vaporization, and measurement of gases like oxygen and carbon dioxide. Furthermore, nonpharmacology-related mathematics skills are essential for dosage calculations and anesthesia management. Mastery of these scientific principles ensures CRNAs can accurately assess, monitor, and adjust anesthesia interventions for optimal patient outcomes.

2. Equipment, Instrumentation, and Technology

Anesthetic delivery systems

Anesthetic delivery systems are essential components of anesthesia practice. These systems ensure the safe and precise administration of anesthetic agents during surgical procedures. These systems also encompass various equipment and devices, including high/low-pressure gas sources, regulators, flow meters, vaporizers, proportioning systems, and safety devices like pressure failure and failsafe mechanisms. While maintaining proper ventilation, anesthetic circuits such as rebreathing (circle system), nonrebreathing, and modified nonrebreathing circuits facilitate the delivery of gases to patients. Moreover, pneumatic and electronic alarm devices provide necessary monitoring and alert systems to ensure patient safety throughout anesthesia administration. During surgery, mastery of these delivery systems is critical for CRNAs to manage anesthesia and safeguard patient well-being effectively.

Airway equipment

Airway equipment is essential to the practice of anesthesia to ensure adequate oxygenation and ventilation during surgical procedures. This equipment contains face masks, laryngoscopes (including rigid, video, and optically enhanced scopes), flexible fiber optic bronchoscopes, endotracheal tubes, and specialized tubes like endobronchial tubes and supraglottic airways such as the Laryngeal Mask Airway (LMA). In addition, tools like intubating stylets, cricothyrotomy kits, and intubation aids like bougies and exchange catheters assist in securing the airway in various clinical scenarios. Understanding and proficiency in utilizing this airway equipment are crucial for CRNAs to effectively manage airway patency and ensure patient safety throughout anesthesia administration.

Monitoring devices

During the administration of anesthesia, monitoring devices are essential tools for nurse anesthetists to conduct a thorough assessment and manage the patient's vital signs and physiological parameters. Central nervous system monitoring involves evoked potentials, intracranial pressure measurement, modified EEG monitors, and cerebral oximetry that facilitates real-time assessment of neurological function and perfusion. Cardiovascular monitoring includes electrocardiography, arterial pressure monitoring, central venous and pulmonary artery pressure monitoring, hemodynamic monitoring, and transesophageal echocardiography to evaluate cardiac function and fluid status. Respiratory monitoring comprises capnography, pulse oximetry, and airway gas analysis, ensuring adequate ventilation and oxygenation. Additionally, peripheral nerve stimulators, temperature monitors, and maternal/fetal monitoring devices offer valuable insights into neuromuscular function, body temperature regulation, and obstetric care during anesthesia. Mastery of these monitoring devices is essential for CRNAs to optimize patient safety and outcomes during surgical procedures.

Patient warming equipment

Patient warming equipment plays a crucial role in maintaining normothermia and preventing perioperative hypothermia, which can lead to adverse outcomes. These devices include fluid/blood warmers, forced air warming devices, heat and moisture exchangers (HME), and radiant warmers. These ensure patient comfort and stability throughout surgical procedures.

Infusion devices

Infusion devices, such as rapid infusers, are essential tools for delivering fluids and medications rapidly and accurately during surgical procedures. These devices help in maintaining hemodynamic stability and optimize patient care.

Imaging and imaging safety

Imaging modalities like ultrasound, fluoroscopy, and radiography are important for guiding interventions and assessing patient anatomy during anesthesia. Understanding imaging safety protocols ensures patient and staff safety during procedures.

3. General Principles of Anesthesia

Ethical considerations

Ethical considerations in anesthesia practice contain principles of beneficence, autonomy, and nonmaleficence which ensure patient rights, safety, and well-being. Further, restriction to research ethics is crucial for conducting ethical research studies, minimizing harm, respecting participant autonomy, and upholding scientific transparency and integrity in anesthesia research endeavors.

Legal issues

Legal issues in anesthesia practice contain a range of topics which include advance healthcare directives, disclosure of errors/injuries, informed consent, legal doctrines, scope of practice, torts, standards of practice, and billing. Understanding these problems is crucial for CRNAs to assure patient rights and safety, steer the legal landscape of healthcare delivery, and sustain compliance with legal and regulatory requirements in their practice.

Safety and wellness

In anesthesia practice, safety and wellness initiatives address crucial problems like provider substance abuse disorder, patient safety issues, and impaired provider concerns. Enforcing wellness initiatives and peer assistance programs helps manage substance abuse issues, foster provider well-being, and maintain a safe environment for patients and healthcare professionals alike.

Preoperative assessment and preparation of patient

Preoperative assessment and preparation include a thorough assessment of the patient's health status, correction of medical conditions, and identification of possible risks to ensure safe administration of anesthesia and surgical outcomes.

Fluid volume assessment and management

Fluid volume assessment and management are important factors of anesthesia care which include fluid and blood component therapy, bloodless medicine procedures like blood salvage devices and hemodilution, and goal-directed fluid management techniques to optimize patient hemodynamics and assure adequate tissue perfusion during surgical procedures.

Positioning

Positioning techniques in anesthesia include optimizing patient positioning for surgical access while minimizing anatomical changes and potential complications, like pressure ulcers, nerve injuries, and poor ventilation or circulation.

Utilization and interpretation of data

In anesthesia, utilization and interpretation of testing data include analyzing lab tests such as activated clotting time and blood gases, as well as diagnostic exams like basic 12-lead ECG interpretation, to ensure patient safety and guide perioperative management decisions.

Airway management

In anesthesia, airway management involves the comprehensive assessment of the airway, employing various techniques, devices, and procedures to secure it safely. Understanding the possible complications and implementing the procedures outlined in the difficult airway algorithm is critical to effectively managing challenging airway scenarios.

Local/regional anesthetics (technique, physiologic alterations, complications)

Local and regional anesthetics are crucial elements of anesthesia practice that offer targeted pain comfort while minimizing systemic effects. Techniques involve understanding anatomy for precise placement, like neuraxial blocks for spinal anesthesia, or peripheral blocks like nerve blocks for extremities. Utilizing ultrasound or nerve stimulator guidance improves safety and accuracy. However, intricacies like local anesthetic systemic toxicity need immediate recognition and management to assure the safety of the patient.

Light, moderate, and deep sedation (monitored anesthesia care)

Light, moderate, and deep sedation, also known as monitored anesthesia care (MAC), provides different consciousness levels during medical procedures while ensuring safety through continuous monitoring and maintaining patient responsiveness.

Total intravenous anesthesia

Total intravenous anesthesia (TIVA) concerns administering all anesthetic agents intravenously, omitting inhaled gases. It offers detailed control over anesthesia depth and is appropriate for different surgical procedures, especially for patients with respiratory concerns.

Pain

Pain involves understanding its physiological, anatomical, pathological, and psychodynamic factors, including chronic and acute presentations. Pain management strategies address chronic and acute pain conditions by utilizing multimodal techniques tailored to individual patient needs.

Enhanced recovery after surgery (ERAS)

Enhanced Recovery After Surgery (ERAS) is a multidisciplinary practice aimed at improving perioperative care to decrease complications, accelerate patient recovery, and enhance outcomes after surgical procedures.

Hypotensive technique and risks

The hypotensive technique involves deliberately lowering blood pressure during surgery to reduce bleeding and improve surgical field visualization. Risks include compromised tissue perfusion, organ damage, and cardiovascular instability if not carefully managed.

Postanesthesia care/respiratory therapy

Postanesthesia care and respiratory therapy include monitoring patients after surgery to ensure safe recovery while focusing on respiratory function. This includes oxygen therapy, airway management, and evaluation for complications such as respiratory depression or airway obstruction.

Infection control

In healthcare settings, infection control involves measures to prevent the spread of infections, including sterilization of equipment, hand hygiene, proper waste disposal, and acting up to standard precautions to reduce the risk of healthcare-associated infections.

Intraoperative fire safety

Intraoperative fire safety protocols include reducing the risk of surgical fire by implementing safety measures, such as ensuring the proper use of electrosurgical equipment, minimizing the concentration of flammable agents, and maintaining a fire-safe environment through adequate ventilation and fire extinguisher availability.

4. Anesthesia for Surgical Procedures and Special Populations

Surgical and diagnostic anesthesia, including management of complications

Surgical and diagnostic anesthesia contains a huge range of procedures in different surgical specialties, each requiring specialized anesthetic management to assure optimal surgical outcomes and patient safety. Anesthetists must tailor their approach to the specific requirements of each patient and procedure, from intra-abdominal surgeries including gastrointestinal, hepatobiliary, and gynecologic procedures to extrathoracic surgeries like breast and plastic/reconstructive surgeries. Cardiac anesthesia addresses open and minimally invasive cardiac procedures, while noncardiac intrathoracic surgery covers conditions of the diaphragm, lungs, esophagus, and mediastinum. Orthopedic procedures, neuroskeletal interventions, and vascular surgeries need precise anesthetic techniques. Perineal and pelvic procedures, non-operating-room anesthesia (NORA) settings, and vascular surgeries further extend the scope of anesthetic practice, in which adaptability and expertise in diverse clinical settings are required. Further, anesthetists may experience robotic/laparoscopic surgeries, organ transplants, burns, trauma cases, and other specialized procedures that emphasize the breadth of anesthesia practice in supporting different surgical interventions.

Anesthesia for special populations

Anesthesia for particular populations requires a critical approach to address the unique anatomic and clinical considerations. Pediatricians demand an understanding of developmental anatomy, pharmacology, and appropriate anesthesia techniques to effectively manage complications. Obstetric anesthesia includes maternal physiology, pharmacology of agents safe for both mother and fetus and management of high-risk conditions such as postpartum hemorrhage. Geriatric patients need attention to age-related anatomical and physiological changes, pharmacological considerations, and techniques to minimize intricacies such as postoperative cognitive dysfunction. Anesthesia for obese individuals includes adjustments for altered anatomy, pharmacology, and special methods such as bariatric anesthesia to reduce perioperative risks. The substance use disorder populations require the management of medication-assisted treatment regimens, pharmacological interactions, and effective pain management strategies while assuring patient safety. Immune-compromised and oncology patients need expertise in anesthesia techniques, pharmacology, and careful perioperative management to optimize outcomes while considering the compromised immune system of the patient.

Duties of the Nurse anesthetists:

- Perform pre-anesthesia assessments and produce anesthesia care plans tailored to the patient's individual needs.

- During surgical procedures, administer anesthesia agents and adjunctive medications.

- Throughout the perioperative period, monitor the patient's vital signs and anesthesia depth.

- During anesthesia administration, manage airways and ensure adequate ventilation.

- Provide pain management interventions including regional anesthesia techniques.

- Respond immediately to intraoperative emergencies and implement suitable interventions.

- To ensure patient safety, collaborate with nurses, surgeons, and other healthcare team members.
- Educate patients and families about postoperative care and anesthesia procedures.
- Document accurately anesthesia-related assessments, interventions, and outcomes.
- Adhere to infection control protocols and maintain a sterile surgical field during procedures.
- Participate in quality improvement initiatives to improve anesthesia care delivery.
- In anesthesia, stay updated with present evidence-based practices and guidelines.
- Manage anesthesia equipment, including maintenance and troubleshooting.
- Provide guidance and support to anesthesia assistants and other team members.
- Assure compliance with regulatory standards and institutional policies related to anesthesia practice.
- Advocate for the safety of a patient and promote a safety culture within the perioperative environment.
- Conduct post-anesthetic evaluations and facilitate patient recovery from anesthesia.
- Cooperate with pain management specialists to optimize postoperative pain control.
- Participate in multidisciplinary rounds and patient care conferences to coordinate perioperative care.
- Engage in professional development activities, including certification maintenance and continuing education.

Conclusion

In conclusion, the study guide for the NBCRNA SEE exam provides a thorough overview of the crucial topics, skills, and responsibilities required of nurse anesthetists. This guide equips CRNA candidates with the knowledge and confidence needed to excel in their profession from understanding the fundamentals of anesthesia practice to mastering advanced techniques and ensuring patient safety. This guide is a valuable resource for CRNAs at every stage of their careers, focusing on continuous learning, professional development, and adherence to standards of excellence.

NBCRNA Self-Evaluation Examination Practice Test

Q1. During anesthesia, what is the primary determinant of myocardial oxygen consumption?

A. Heart rate

B. Blood pressure

C. Cardiac contractility

D. Coronary artery diameter

Q2. Which factor significantly contributes to coronary perfusion pressure during cardiopulmonary resuscitation (CPR)?

A. Diastolic blood pressure

B. Mean arterial pressure

C. Systolic blood pressure

D. Chest compression depth

Q3. For increased airway resistance, which respiratory parameter is most indicative?

A. Decreased tidal volume

B. Increased respiratory rate

C. Decreased expiratory flow rate

D. Increased inspiratory capacity

Q4. Considering the following, what is the primary determinant of alveolar ventilation?

A. Respiratory rate

B. Tidal volume

C. Dead space ventilation

D. Alveolar dead space

Q5. In the central nervous system, which neurotransmitter is primarily responsible for inhibiting neuronal activity?

A. Dopamine

B. Acetylcholine

C. Gamma-aminobutyric acid (GABA)

D. Glutamate

Q6. Which region of the brain is most likely to result in deficits in voluntary motor control and coordination due to damage?

A. Cerebellum

B. Medulla oblongata

C. Hypothalamus

D. Frontal lobe

Q7. For transmitting forces between muscles and bones in the human body, which anatomical structure is responsible?

A. Ligament

B. Tendon

C. Cartilage

D. Synovium

Q8. For promoting glycogen breakdown in the liver, which hormone regulates blood glucose levels?

A. Insulin

B. Glucagon

C. Cortisol

D. Thyroxine

Q9. What is the primary function of the renal tubules in the nephron considering the following?

A. Filtration of blood

B. Reabsorption of water and nutrients

C. Production of urine

D. Regulation of blood pressure

Q10. Which hormone is responsible for stimulating erythropoiesis in response to hypoxia?

A. Insulin

B. Thyroid hormone

C. Erythropoietin

D. Parathyroid hormone

Q11. Within the stomach, which hormone stimulates the secretion of hydrochloric acid and pepsinogen?

A. Insulin

B. Glucagon

C. Gastrin

D. Secretin

Q12. In the immune system, which cells are responsible for antibody production?

A. T cells

B. B cells

C. Natural killer cells

D. Macrophages

Q13. What is the MOST specific biochemical marker for myocardial injury? (Select 2).

A. Creatine kinase-MB (CK-MB)

B. Troponin I

C. Myoglobin

D. Lactate dehydrogenase (LDH)

Q14. Which valvular heart disease is characterized by a diastolic murmur and a widened pulse pressure? (Select 2)

A. Aortic regurgitation

B. Aortic stenosis

C. Mitral regurgitation

D. Mitral stenosis

Q15. Which respiratory obstructive disease is characterized by reversible airflow limitation and airway inflammation? (Select 2)

A. Asthma

B. Chronic bronchitis

C. Emphysema

D. Bronchiectasis

Q16. Which neurodegenerative disease is characterized by the presence of Lewy bodies and affects both motor and cognitive functions? (Select 2)

A. Parkinson's disease

B. Alzheimer's disease

C. Huntington's disease

D. Amyotrophic lateral sclerosis

Q17. During anesthesia induction, which metabolic abnormality increases the risk of malignant hyperthermia? (Select 2)

A. Hyperkalemia

B. Hypocalcemia

C. Hypernatremia

D. Hyperthermia

Q18. For regulating calcium levels in the blood and bone, which hormone is responsible? (Select 2)

A. Thyroid-stimulating hormone (TSH)

B. Parathyroid hormone (PTH)

C. Thyroxine (T4)

D. Calcitonin

Q19. Which infectious disease primarily affects the liver and is caused by the hepatitis B virus? (Select 2)

A. Hepatitis A

B. Hepatitis B

C. Hepatitis C

D. Hepatitis E

Q20. Which condition is characterized by glomerular inflammation, hematuria, proteinuria, and often hypertension? (Select 2)

A. IgA nephropathy

B. Nephrotic syndrome

C. Acute tubular necrosis

D. Alport syndrome

Q21. What kind of anemia exhibits target cells and increased hemoglobin F levels? (Select 2)

A. Thalassemia

B. Sickle cell anemia

C. Iron deficiency anemia

D. Hemolytic anemia

Q22. Which gastrointestinal disorder exhibits the backward flow of stomach acid into the esophagus and regurgitation of food? (Select 2)

A. Gastroesophageal reflux disease (GERD)

B. Achalasia

C. Barrett's esophagus

D. Hiatal hernia

Q23. What medical condition involves a weakened immune system, leading to susceptibility to opportunistic infections and certain types of cancers? (Select 2)

A. HIV/AIDS

B. Tuberculosis

C. Hepatitis B

D. Malaria

Q24. Which is a characteristic feature of cancer cells among the following? (Select 2)

A. Uncontrolled cell growth

B. Decreased mutation rate

C. Enhanced apoptosis

D. Restored cell cycle regulation

Q25. Which inhalation anesthetics exhibit the highest blood/gas partition coefficients? (Select 3)

A. Nitrous oxide

B. Sevoflurane

C. Desflurane

D. Isoflurane

E. Halothane

F. Xenon

Q26. At the nicotinic acetylcholine receptor, which neuromuscular blocking agent acts as a competitive antagonist? (Select 3)

A. Pancuronium

B. Vecuronium

C. Rocuronium

D. Succinylcholine

E. Atracurium

F. Cisatracurium

Q27. Among the options, which local anesthetic primarily blocks sodium channels and is commonly administered for spinal anesthesia? (Select 3)

A. Bupivacaine

B. Lidocaine

C. Procaine

D. Ropivacaine

E. Tetracaine

F. Mepivacaine

Q28. For local anesthetic systemic toxicity (LAST) and exerts its effects by changing lipid solubility, which pharmacological intervention is used as an antidote? (Select 3)

A. Intravenous calcium gluconate

B. Intravenous bicarbonate

C. Lipid emulsion therapy

D. Intravenous neostigmine

E. Intravenous atropine

F. Intravenous dantrolene

Q29. For prolonging the duration of sensory blockade, which pharmacological agents are commonly used as adjuncts in regional anesthesia? (Select 3)

A. Epinephrine

B. Clonidine

C. Dexmedetomidine

D. Dexamethasone

E. Buprenorphine

F. Magnesium sulfate

Q30. Among pharmacological options used in anesthesia, which are considered anticholinergics or cholinergic agonists? (Select 3)

A. Atropine

B. Glycopyrrolate

C. Neostigmine

D. Edrophonium

E. Bethanechol

F. Physostigmine

Q31. Which medications used in anesthesia are classified as non-opioid analgesics? (Select 3)

A. Acetaminophen

B. Nonsteroidal anti-inflammatory drugs (NSAIDs)

C. Ketamine

D. Gabapentin

E. Lidocaine

F. Tramadol

Q32. In anesthesia practice, which medications are commonly used as bronchodilators? (Select 3)

A. Albuterol

B. Ipratropium

C. Theophylline

D. Formoterol

E. Salmeterol

F. Aclidinium

Q33. Which effects are associated with prostaglandin administration? (Select 3)

A. Vasodilation

B. Bronchoconstriction

C. Increased gastric acid secretion

D. Uterine contraction

E. Platelet aggregation inhibition

F. Decreased renal blood flow

Q34. Which effects are associated with histamine receptor antagonists? (Select 3)

A. Decreased gastric acid secretion

B. Prevention of gastric ulcers

C. Treatment of gastroesophageal reflux disease

D. Relief of allergic symptoms

E. Reduction of symptoms associated with peptic ulcers

F. Prevention of motion sickness

Q35. Which effects are associated with insulin administration? (Select 3)

A. Promotion of glucose uptake by cells

B. Inhibition of hepatic glucose production

C. Stimulation of glycogen synthesis

D. Enhancement of lipolysis

E. Facilitation of protein synthesis

F. Inhibition of ketogenesis

Q36. What kind of mechanisms are involved in the action of hypoglycemic medications? (Select 3)

A. Promotion of insulin release from pancreatic beta cells

B. Enhancement of insulin sensitivity in peripheral tissues

C. Inhibition of hepatic glucose production

D. Stimulation of glucose uptake by cells

E. Delay of carbohydrate absorption in the gastrointestinal tract

F. Inhibition of glucagon secretion

Q37. The concentration of a solution which represents the number of moles of solute dissolved per liter of solution is typically expressed in _____.

Q38. The products formed in a neutralization reaction between hydrochloric acid (HCl) and sodium hydroxide (NaOH) are sodium chloride (NaCl) and _____.

Q39. Glucose undergoes _____ to produce carbon dioxide, water, and ATP energy in the cellular respiration process.

Q40. Glucose is broken down through the process of __ to produce ATP energy and carbon dioxide during cellular metabolism.

Q41. Signal transduction often involves the binding of a ligand to a _____ on the cell membrane in cellular mechanisms of action, initiating intracellular signaling cascades.

Q42. Agonists bind to receptors and initiate a response, during drug-receptor interaction, while _____ bind to receptors and block agonist action without eliciting a response.

Q43. The unit of measurement for length is _____ in the International System of Units (SI).

Q44. At constant temperature, the pressure of a gas is _____ proportional to its volume, according to Boyle's law.

Q45. The rate of diffusion of a gas across a membrane is _____ proportional to the surface area and the concentration gradient, according to Fick's law of diffusion.

Q46. In the context of fluid dynamics, Poiseuille's law states that the flow rate of a fluid through a cylindrical tube is _____ proportional to the pressure gradient and the fourth power of the radius.

Q47. In the context of electrical safety, using insulated tools and equipment and ensuring that all circuits are properly _____ is the most effective way to prevent electrical shock.

Q48. The formula: dose = concentration × _____ × weight is used to calculate the amount of drug to administer.

Q49. In anesthesia delivery systems, which gas source typically provides gases at higher pressures?

A) Oxygen concentrator

B) Cylinder gases

C) Pipeline gases

D) Liquid oxygen

Q50. Which component of an anesthetic delivery system ensures the safety of gas for patient use by regulating its pressure upon entry into the system?

A) Vaporizer

B) Flowmeter

C) Regulator

D) Manifold

Q51. Which component of an anesthetic delivery system controls the rate of gas flow by adjusting the size of an orifice through which the gas passes?

A) Vaporizer

B) Flowmeter

C) Valve

D) Float

Q52. During anesthesia induction, which anesthetic delivery system's component is responsible for vaporizing liquid anesthetic agents into a precise concentration for inhalation?

A) Flowmeter

B) Vaporizer

C) Valve

D) Filter

Q53. Which component's responsibility is to accurately mix the desired concentrations of oxygen and volatile anesthetic agents, in anesthetic delivery systems?

A) Vaporizer

B) Flowmeter

C) Proportioning system

D) Breathing circuit

Q54. In the event of a loss of gas pressure, which component of an anesthetic delivery system is designed to prevent the delivery of anesthetic gases?

A) Vaporizer

B) Flowmeter

C) Proportioning system

D) Pressure failure safety device

Q55. What role does the proportioning system play in anesthetic delivery systems?

A) Ensuring accurate gas flow rates

B) Monitoring patient vital signs

C) Regulating the concentration of anesthetic gases

D) Preventing contamination of anesthesia equipment

Q56. Despite changes in compliance or resistance, which function of the ventilator ensures that the delivered tidal volume matches the set volume?

A) Pressure control

B) Volume control

C) Pressure support

D) Dual control

Q57. To remove exhaled carbon dioxide from the breathing circuit, which compound is commonly used as a carbon dioxide absorbent in anesthesia machines?

A) Soda lime

B) Zeolite

C) Silica gel

D) Calcium sulfate

Q58. In a circle anesthesia system, what is the primary function of the reservoir bag?

A) Store anesthetic gases

B) Provide a visual indicator of patient ventilation

C) Absorb exhaled carbon dioxide

D) Facilitate manual ventilation

Q59. What is a primary advantage of using a non-rebreathing anesthesia circuit?

A) Allows for the rebreathing of exhaled gases

B) Minimizes the risk of carbon dioxide buildup

C) Requires a lower fresh gas flow rate

D) Enhances humidity and warmth of inspired gases

Q60. In anesthetic delivery systems, what is the primary purpose of pneumatic and electronic alarm devices?

A) To regulate the flow of anesthetic gases

B) To provide audible and visual alerts for abnormal conditions

C) To monitor patient vital signs during anesthesia

D) To ensure proper waste gas scavenging

Q61. In the context of anesthesia, which of the following are advantages of using face masks? (Select 2)

A) Ability to deliver high concentrations of oxygen

B) Provides a tight seal over the patient's nose and mouth

C) Allows for easy visualization of the patient's airway

D) Minimizes the risk of aerosolization of infectious agents

Q62. During intubation, which of the following are advantages of using a laryngoscope? (Select 2)

A) Provides direct visualization of the vocal cords

B) Facilitates passage of the endotracheal tube into the trachea

C) Allows for continuous monitoring of end-tidal CO2

D) Assists in confirming proper tube placement using capnography

Q63. Which of the following are important considerations when using a flexible fiberoptic bronchoscope for intubation? (Select 2)

A) Ability to navigate through anatomical structures

B) Limited visibility due to fogging of the lens

C) Use of topical anesthesia to minimize patient discomfort

D) Risk of bronchospasm in patients with reactive airway disease

Q64. For an endotracheal tube cuff, which of the following characteristics are essential? (Select 2)

A. Low volume, high pressure

B. High volume, low pressure

C. High volume, high pressure

D. Low volume, low pressure

Q65. When selecting an appropriate double-lumen endobronchial tube, which of the following characteristics are crucial? (Select 2)

A. Size of the distal cuff

B. Length of the tracheal portion

C. Placement of the bronchial lumen

D. Diameter of the carinal hook

Q66. Which factors should be considered when selecting a bronchial blocker for lung isolation? (Select 2)

A. Size of the blocker

B. Length of the blocker

C. Positioning of the blocker

D. Diameter of the bronchial lumen

Q67. Which factors should be considered when selecting an oral airway? (Select 2)

A. Length of the airway

B. Diameter of the airway

C. Flexibility of the airway

D. Positioning of the patient

Q68. Which factors should be considered when selecting a nasal airway? (Select 2)

A. Size of the airway

B. Length of the airway

C. Flexibility of the airway

D. Positioning of the patient

Q69. Which factors should be considered when selecting a tracheostomy tube? (Select 2)

A. Inner diameter of the tube

B. Length of the tube

C. Presence of cuff

D. Material of the tube

Q70. What should be assessed to confirm proper placement when using a supraglottic airway device such as the LMA? (Select 2)

A. Bilateral chest rise

B. Presence of breath sounds in the epigastrium

C. Symmetrical chest movement

D. Condensation in the device

Q71. What steps are essential before advancing the endotracheal tube when using an intubating supraglottic airway device? (Select 2)

A. Confirming bilateral chest rise

B. Ensuring adequate ventilation

C. Assessing for fogging in the tube

D. Verifying correct placement with capnography

Q72. In airway management, which of the following are advantages of jet ventilation? (Select 2)

A. Decreased risk of barotrauma

B. Improved surgical exposure

C. Enhanced carbon dioxide elimination

D. Lower incidence of air trapping

Q73. In difficult airway management, what are the advantages of using intubating stylets? (Select 3)

A. Facilitation of endotracheal tube placement

B. Improved visualization of the glottic opening

C. Enhanced maneuverability in restricted airways

D. Decreased risk of dental trauma

E. Swift passage through anatomical obstructions

F. Minimization of soft tissue injury

Q74. In emergency airway management, what are the primary indications for performing a cricothyrotomy? (Select 3)

A. Failed endotracheal intubation

B. Severe upper airway obstruction

C. Need for urgent airway access

D. Inability to ventilate with mask ventilation

E. Anticipated difficult airway due to trauma

F. Acute laryngeal edema compromising airway

Q75. In difficult airway management, which of the following are examples of intubation aids commonly used? (Select 3)

A. Endotracheal tube introducer

B. Gum elastic bougie

C. Airway exchange catheter

D. Stylet

E. Laryngeal mask airway

F. Video laryngoscope

Q76. To assess central nervous system function through evoked potentials, which monitoring device is commonly used? (Select 3)

A. Pulse oximeter

B. Capnograph

C. Electroencephalogram (EEG)

D. Near-infrared spectroscopy (NIRS)

E. Bispectral index monitor (BIS)

F. Somatosensory evoked potential (SSEP) monitor

Q77. In neurosurgical patients, which monitoring device is commonly used to directly measure intracranial pressure? (Select 3)

A. Pulmonary artery catheter

B. Transesophageal echocardiography probe

C. Intracranial pressure (ICP) monitor

D. Transcutaneous oxygen saturation monitor

E. Esophageal stethoscope

F. Pulse contour cardiac output (PiCCO) monitor

Q78. When analyzing electroencephalographic activity to assess cerebral function, which monitoring device can be modified to monitor depth of anesthesia? (Select 3)

A. Pulse oximeter

B. Bispectral Index (BIS) monitor

C. Capnograph

D. Transesophageal echocardiography probe

E. Intracranial pressure (ICP) monitor

F. Near-infrared spectroscopy (NIRS) monitor

Q79. Which monitoring device is used to assess neuromuscular blockade and guide the titration of muscle relaxants during anesthesia? (Select 3)

A. Train-of-four (TOF) monitor

B. Capnograph

C. Bispectral Index (BIS) monitor

D. Peripheral nerve stimulator

E. Pulse oximeter

F. End-tidal anesthetic gas monitor

Q80. What leads are commonly part of a standard 3-lead electrocardiogram (ECG)? (Select 3)

A. Lead I, Lead II, Lead III

B. Lead V1, Lead V2, Lead V3

C. Lead aVR, Lead aVL, Lead aVF

D. Lead aVR, Lead V1, Lead V5

E. Lead V1, Lead V4, Lead V6

F. Lead II, Lead III, Lead aVF

Q81. During the anesthesia, which monitoring device is commonly used for continuous arterial pressure monitoring? (Select 3)

A. Pulse oximeter

B. Continuous cardiac output monitor

C. Arterial line

D. Central venous catheter

E. Transesophageal echocardiography probe

F. Capnograph

Q82. In anesthetized patients, which noninvasive monitoring device is commonly used to assess blood pressure? (Select 3)

A. Echocardiogram

B. Doppler ultrasound

C. Continuous cardiac output monitor

D. Oscillometric blood pressure cuff

E. Transesophageal echocardiography probe

F. Capnograph

Q83. A nurse anesthetist administers a medication to a patient, but due to a calculation error, the dosage exceeds the prescribed limit. What legal principle is implicated in this situation? (Select 3.)

A. Respondeat superior

B. Informed consent

C. Duty of care

D. Contributory negligence

E. Vicarious liability

F. Disclosure of errors/injuries

Q84. In anesthetized patients, which monitoring device is commonly used to assess central venous pressure? (Select 3)

A. Pulse oximeter

B. Capnograph

C. Arterial line transducer

D. Central venous catheter

E. Doppler ultrasound

F. Esophageal stethoscope

Q85. To assess pulmonary artery pressure and mixed venous oxygen saturation (SvO2) in critically ill patients, which monitoring device is commonly used? (Select 3)

A. Pulse oximeter

B. Capnograph

C. Transesophageal echocardiography

D. Pulmonary artery catheter with fiberoptic sensor

E. Swan-Ganz catheter

F. Transcutaneous oxygen saturation monitor

Q86. Which monitoring devices provide continuous assessment of stroke volume, systemic vascular resistance, cardiac output, and other hemodynamic parameters? (Select 3)

A. Electrocardiogram (ECG)

B. Transesophageal echocardiography (TEE)

C. Arterial line waveform analysis

D. Pulmonary artery catheter (PAC)

E. Non-invasive blood pressure cuff

F. Impedance cardiography

Q87. A _____ echocardiogram provides real-time images of cardiac structures and function during cardiac surgery, aiding in the assessment of valvular function, ventricular contractility, and intracardiac volumes.

Q88. In exhaled breath, capnography is the measurement of _____, providing continuous monitoring of ventilation adequacy and early detection of airway compromise or respiratory distress.

Q89. Airway gas analysis, such as the measurement of _____, provides crucial information on pulmonary gas exchange, during anesthesia, it aids in the assessment of ventilation and oxygenation status.

Q90. To assess neuromuscular blockade during anesthesia by delivering _____ impulses to the peripheral nerve the peripheral nerve stimulator is used, eliciting a response in the corresponding muscle.

Q91. To maintain patient safety and homeostasis, temperature monitoring during anesthesia is crucial. Commonly used devices include tympanic membrane probes, esophageal probes, and _____ probes.

Q92. In patients receiving large-volume infusions, during perioperative care, the use of fluid/blood warmers helps prevent _____ by maintaining normothermia.

Q93. To prevent _____ and maintain normothermia in surgical patients, forced air warming devices are commonly used intraoperatively, reducing the risk of perioperative complications related to hypothermia.

Q94. To deliver large volumes of fluids and blood products _____, rapid infusers are utilized intraoperatively, ensuring rapid restoration of intravascular volume in critically ill or hemorrhaging patients.

Q95. In anesthesia, ultrasound is commonly used for real-time visualization of anatomical structures such as nerves vessels, and the airway, enhancing procedural accuracy and _____.

Q96. To visualize structures within the body, fluoroscopy is a real-time imaging technique that uses X-rays, aiding in procedures such as _____.

Q97. Which principle emphasizes respecting a patient's right to make informed decisions about their care in ethical considerations for anesthesia practice?

A. Autonomy

B. Beneficence

C. Nonmalfeasance

D. Justice

Q98. Which action aligns with promoting the patient's well-being, when considering beneficence in anesthesia practice?

A. Withholding necessary information

B. Prioritizing personal beliefs over patient preferences

C. Providing optimal pain management

D. Disregarding informed consent

Q99. Which principle emphasizes the requirement to obtain voluntary, informed consent from participants in the context of research ethics?

A. Autonomy

B. Beneficence

C. Nonmaleficence

D. Justice

Q100. In research ethics, which principle guides researchers to maximize benefits and minimize harm to research participants?

A. Autonomy

B. Beneficence

C. Nonmaleficence

D. Justice

Q101. Which legal principle ensures that an anesthetist respects a patient's previously stated wishes about end-of-life care in the context of Advance Healthcare Directives? (Select 2.)

A. Autonomy protection

B. Beneficence obligation

C. Nonmaleficence mandate

D. Veracity commitment

Q102. Which legal documents empower a designated individual to make medical decisions for an incapacitated patient when implementing Advance Healthcare Directives? (Select 2.)

A. Living will

B. Durable power of attorney for healthcare

C. Informed consent form

D. Physician's order for life-sustaining treatment (POLST)

Q103. For obtaining valid informed consent before administering anesthesia, which element is essential in the context of legal considerations? (Select 2.)

A. Patient's age

B. Anesthesia provider's preference

C. Family member's opinion

D. Detailed explanation of risks and benefits

Q104. For demonstrating the informed consent process, which documentation is crucial when addressing legal aspects of informed consent? (Select 2.)

A. Anesthesia provider's notes

B. Family member's signature

C. Detailed anesthesia equipment list

D. Witnessed patient refusal form

Q105. A nurse anesthetist administers a medication to a patient, but the dosage exceeds the prescribed limit due to a calculation error. In this situation, which of the following principles is implicated? (Select 3.)

A. Respondeat superior

B. Informed consent

C. Duty of care

D. Contributory negligence

E. Vicarious liability

F. Disclosure of errors/injuries

Q106. Before obtaining consent, which principle emphasizes the duty to disclose all relevant information to the patient in the context of legal doctrines related to anesthesia practice? (Select 3.)

A. Res ipsa loquitur

B. Informed consent

C. Respondeat superior

D. Statute of limitations

E. Assumption of risk

F. Good Samaritan law

Q107. Which legal concept is most relevant, when a patient undergoing surgery experiences an unexpected allergic reaction to a medication, resulting in harm? (Select 3.)

A. Res ipsa loquitur

B. Contributory negligence

C. Strict liability

D. Informed consent

E. Standard of care

F. Comparative negligence

Q108. Which of the following activities falls within the nurse anesthetist's professional responsibilities in the context of legal issues and scope of practice? (Select 2.)

A. Administering blood transfusions

B. Performing surgical procedures

C. Diagnosing medical conditions

D. Interpreting radiological images

E. Prescribing medications

F. Providing postoperative pain management

Q109. _____ defines the scope of practice for nurse anesthetists, outlining the responsibilities and boundaries within which they must operate.

Q110. To ensure ethical and legal practice in anesthesia care, nurse anesthetists must be aware of and comply with the _____ guidelines.

Q111. Proper documentation of anesthesia services is crucial for billing accuracy. To reflect the specific anesthesia procedures performed in the billing process, it is essential to include the _____ codes.

Q112. When billing for services rendered, anesthesia providers must adhere to legal guidelines. Failure to document medical necessity may result in potential legal scrutiny and _____ reimbursement.

Q113. If a certified registered nurse anesthetist (CRNA) suspects a colleague is struggling with substance abuse, what is the most appropriate action?

A. Ignore the concern to avoid conflict.

B. Report anonymously to hospital administration.

C. Confront the colleague directly.

D. Seek guidance from a professional support program.

Q114. What organizational intervention promotes a culture of safety and wellness, when addressing substance abuse among anesthesia providers?

A. Implementing random drug testing.

B. Creating an environment of fear and punishment.

C. Offering confidential counseling services.

D. Encouraging colleagues to gossip about suspicions.

Q115. Which factor is MOST critical for ensuring patient safety in the administration of anesthesia, during preoperative assessment?

A. Age and gender considerations.

B. Allergies and sensitivities.

C. Past medical history.

D. Recent dietary habits.

Q116. What measure should be prioritized to minimize the risk of medication errors during anesthesia induction, in the context of patient safety?

A. Double-checking drug labels with a colleague.

B. Memorizing drug dosages for common procedures.

C. Relying solely on electronic medication records.

D. Administering medications quickly to save time.

Q117. What immediate action should be taken to prioritize patient safety, when a nurse anesthetist encounters a colleague showing signs of impaired cognitive function during a surgical procedure? (Select 2.)

A. Administer a cholinesterase inhibitor.

B. Increase the depth of anesthesia.

C. Notify the supervisor and relieve the impaired provider.

D. Implement a sedation protocol.

Q118. Which factors contribute to an effective peer monitoring system for anesthesia providers, in the context of ensuring wellness and safety? (Select 2.)

A. Regular assessment of cognitive and psychomotor skills.

B. Encouraging competition among colleagues.

C. Relying solely on self-assessment.

D. Ignoring subtle changes in behavior.

Q119. Which activity is most effective for reducing stress and promoting mental well-being, in the context of wellness initiatives for nurse anesthetists? (Select 2.)

A. Weekly group therapy sessions

B. Individual mindfulness meditation

C. Mandatory overtime shifts

D. Monthly peer assistance workshops

Q120. In promoting safety and wellness among nurse anesthetists, what specific role can peer assistance programs play? (Select 2.)

A. Providing financial incentives for overtime

B. Offering counseling and support for substance abuse

C. Mandating extended work hours

D. Conducting surprise evaluations for performance

Q121. When assessing a patient with severe aortic stenosis preoperatively, what is the primary concern?

A. Bradycardia

B. Hypertension

C. Tachycardia

D. Hypotension

E. Fluid overload

F. Increased afterload

Q122. Which interventions are crucial for minimizing perioperative complications, when preparing a patient with chronic obstructive pulmonary disease (COPD) for surgery? (Select 3.)

A. Bronchodilator therapy

B. Smoking cessation counseling

C. Chest physiotherapy

D. Incentive spirometry

E. Preoperative antibiotic prophylaxis

F. Continuous positive airway pressure (CPAP) at night

Q123. Which indicator is most reliable for assessing intravascular volume status in a critically ill patient, in the context of fluid volume assessment? (Select 3.)

A. Central venous pressure (CVP)

B. Urine output

C. Serum lactate levels

D. Pulmonary artery wedge pressure (PAWP)

E. Serum creatinine

F. Blood urea nitrogen (BUN)

Q124. Which fluid replacement strategy has been shown to improve outcomes, when considering fluid therapy in a patient with septic shock? (Select 3.)

A. Hypertonic saline solution

B. Albumin solution

C. Crystalloid solution

D. Hydroxyethyl starch solution

E. Plasma expander solution

F. Gelatin solution

Q125. In patients undergoing bloodless medicine procedures, what is a primary consideration for fluid volume assessment and management? (Select 3.)

A. Platelet count monitoring

B. Crystalloid boluses

C. Administration of packed red blood cells

D. Hemostatic agent infusion

E. Use of blood salvage devices

F. Hemodilution techniques

Q126. Which interventions contribute to minimizing the need for allogeneic blood transfusion during surgery, in the context of bloodless medicine? (Select 3.)

A. Administration of fresh frozen plasma

B. Aggressive platelet transfusions

C. Preoperative iron supplementation

D. Intraoperative cell salvage

E. Rapid infusion of coagulation factors

F. Routine use of vasopressors

Q127. To improve tissue perfusion goal-directed fluid management involves optimizing cardiac output, often monitored using _____.

Q128. The primary parameter used to guide fluid administration is ____ during goal-directed fluid management.

Q129. To prevent complications, massive transfusion protocol implementation requires continuous ____

Q130. Which laboratory test is commonly used to evaluate hemostasis and guide transfusion decisions, in the context of fluid volume assessment?

A. Prothrombin Time (PT)

B. Activated Partial Thromboplastin Time (aPTT)

C. Platelet Count

D. Serum Creatinine

Q131. What does Thromboelastography (TEG) primarily assess, aiding in the optimization of coagulation support, during perioperative fluid management?

A. Platelet function

B. Serum electrolytes

C. Renal function

D. Cardiac output

Q132. What is the recommended positioning for a patient with a history of myotonic dystrophy, during anesthetic management?

A. Supine with legs elevated.

B. Prone with neck flexed.

C. Lithotomy with arms abducted.

D. Lateral decubitus with head elevated.

Q133. Which technique is commonly employed to avoid compression of the ulnar nerve and subsequent complications, when positioning a patient for anesthesia?

A. Padding the elbows.

B. Utilizing a gel mattress.

C. Elevating the legs.

D. Placing arms on arm boards.

Q134. What physiological alteration should be monitored closely to prevent complications, during prone positioning for surgery? (Select 2.)

A. Increased heart rate

B. Decreased tidal volume

C. Elevated blood pressure

D. Hypercapnia

Q135. Which hemodynamic changes should be anticipated, in a patient undergoing Trendelenburg positioning? (Select 2.)

A. Increased preload

B. Decreased afterload

C. Elevated heart rate

D. Reduced cardiac contractility

Q136. During surgery, which complications are associated with the prone positioning of a patient? (Select 2.)

A. Ocular compression

B. Airway obstruction

C. Peripheral nerve injury

D. Increased risk of venous thromboembolism

Q137. In anesthesia, what are potential complications related to the lithotomy position? (Select 2.)

A. Nerve injury

B. Impaired circulation to lower extremities

C. Increased risk of atelectasis

D. Elevated intracranial pressure

Q138. Which laboratory test is MOST likely to provide additional valuable information, when an elevated serum lactate level is detected in the preoperative assessment of a patient scheduled for major surgery? (Select 3.)

A. Complete Blood Count (CBC)

B. Arterial Blood Gas (ABG)

C. Activated Clotting Time (ACT)

D. Liver Function Tests (LFTs)

E. Serum Electrolytes

F. Creatinine Clearance

Q139. Which combination of laboratory tests is MOST appropriate for assessing both primary and secondary hemostasis, when a patient with a history of von Willebrand disease is scheduled for elective surgery? (Select 3.)

A. Platelet count, Prothrombin Time (PT), D-dimer

B. Activated Clotting Time (ACT), Fibrinogen, Bleeding Time

C. Platelet Function Assay, International Normalized Ratio (INR), Thrombin Time

D. von Willebrand Factor Antigen, Platelet count, Activated Partial Thromboplastin Time (aPTT)

E. Factor VIII assay, Fibrinogen, Platelet Function Assay

F. D-dimer, Activated Partial Thromboplastin Time (aPTT), Platelet count

Q140. In a patient undergoing surgery, an abnormal elevation in the ST segment of a 12-lead ECG is most indicative of: (Select 3.)

A. Hypokalemia

B. Hypercalcemia

C. Myocardial ischemia

D. Atrial fibrillation

E. Left bundle-branch block

F. Ventricular tachycardia

Q141. Which finding on a preoperative chest X-ray is most concerning for the potential development of postoperative atelectasis, when interpreting a diagnostic exam? (Select 3.)

A. Hyperinflated lungs

B. Prominent pulmonary vasculature

C. Elevated hemidiaphragm

D. Subsegmental atelectasis

E. Pleural effusion

F. Widened mediastinum

Q142. The Mallampati classification evaluates _____ visibility and predicts ease of intubation, during airway assessment.

Q143. The thyromental distance is measured from the _____ to the chin. It helps assess airway patency.

Q144. The technique that involves lifting the mandible to open the oropharyngeal space is known as _____ when considering airway management.

Q145. The device commonly used to secure the endotracheal tube and prevent accidental extubation is called a _____ in airway procedures.

Q146. What complication may arise from improper positioning of the endotracheal tube cuff, during airway management?

A. Esophageal intubation

B. Subglottic stenosis

C. Hypopharyngeal rupture

D. Tracheal malacia

Q147. What airway device is often preferred to minimize complications, when utilizing rapid sequence induction for a patient with a known difficult airway?

A. Laryngeal mask airway (LMA)

B. Endotracheal tube (ETT)

C. Combitube

D. King LT-D airway

Q148. Which airway device is specifically designed for use in patients with limited mouth opening, in the context of difficult airway management?

A. Laryngeal Mask Airway (LMA)

B. Bougie

C. GlideScope

D. Cricothyrotomy Kit

Q149. Which induction agent is preferred due to its rapid onset and short duration of action, when encountering a difficult airway during induction?

A. Etomidate

B. Propofol

C. Ketamine

D. Midazolam

Q150. When administering a local anesthetic for an axillary nerve block, what anatomical consideration is crucial? (Select 2.)

A. Proximity to the brachial plexus

B. Location of the ulnar nerve

C. Muscular innervation in the forearm

D. Connection to the radial artery

Q151. Which anatomical landmark is crucial for avoiding inadvertent dural puncture, during a lumbar epidural placement? (Select 2.)

A. Spinous process

B. Intervertebral foramen

C. Ligamentum flavum

D. Transverse process

Q152. In regional anesthesia, what is a potential complication associated with local anesthetic infiltration? (Select 2.)

A. Local tissue necrosis

B. Increased cardiac output

C. Elevated blood pressure

D. Bradycardia

Q153. In local anesthetic solutions during infiltration, what physiological alteration is most likely associated with the use of epinephrine in regional anesthesia? (Select 2.)

A. Increased duration of action

B. Reduced vasoconstriction

C. Enhanced nerve blockade

D. Lowered blood pressure

Q154. In the oral cavity, which of the following local anesthetic agents is commonly used topically for mucosal anesthesia? (Select 3.)

A. Lidocaine

B. Bupivacaine

C. Tetracaine

D. Procaine

E. Benzocaine

F. Ropivacaine

Q155. During neuraxial block placement, a common complication associated with unintentional vascular puncture is: (Select 3.)

A. Hypotension

B. Paresthesia

C. Hematoma formation

D. Bradycardia

E. Nausea

F. Infection

Q156. Which of the following complications are associated with continuous peripheral nerve block catheters? (Select 3.)

A. Hematoma formation

B. Local anesthetic systemic toxicity

C. Catheter dislodgement

D. Nerve injury

E. Allergic reaction

F. Infection

Q157. Which local anesthetic agent is commonly associated with a risk of systemic toxicity, manifesting as central nervous system excitation followed by depression? (Select 3.)

A. Bupivacaine

B. Lidocaine

C. Mepivacaine

D. Ropivacaine

E. Procaine

F. Articaine

Q158. Local anesthetics are commonly combined with _____ to enhance their duration and improve postoperative pain management.

Q159. The needle is inserted _____ to avoid inadvertent globe penetration when performing a retrobulbar block for ophthalmic surgery.

Q160. By blocking _____ channels, and inhibiting nerve impulse conduction, local anesthetics exert their effects.

Q161. In the event of suspected local anesthetic systemic toxicity, administer _____ as a specific antidote.

Q162. Which sedative agent is commonly used in monitored anesthesia care for light sedation due to its rapid onset and short duration of action?

A. Propofol

B. Midazolam

C. Dexmedetomidine

D. Ketamine

Q163. In chronic pain management, what psychosocial factors play an important role in influencing pain perception? (Select 2.)

A. Anxiety

B. Depression

C. Euphoria

D. Apathy

Q164. When providing deep sedation in monitored anesthesia care, which medication without respiratory depression is preferred for its analgesic and sedative properties?

A. Fentanyl

B. Remifentanil

C. Morphine

D. Hydromorphone

Q165. For total intravenous anesthesia (TIVA), which pharmacokinetic parameter of propofol makes it suitable?

A. High lipid solubility

B. Long elimination half-life

C. Slow onset of action

D. Minimal protein binding

Q166. In total intravenous anesthesia (TIVA), what is the primary advantage of using remifentanil?

A. Long duration of action

B. Accumulation in fatty tissues

C. Non-metabolism by esterases

D. Slow onset of action

Q167. In the central nervous system, which neurotransmitter is primarily responsible for pain modulation? (Select 2.)

A. Serotonin

B. Dopamine

C. Glutamate

D. Endorphins

Q168. Which analgesic is commonly used for acute pain management in the postoperative period? (Select 2.)

A. Morphine

B. Ibuprofen

C. Gabapentin

D. Lidocaine

Q169. In patients with neuropathic pain, which pharmacological agent is most often indicated for chronic pain management? (Select 2.)

A. Tramadol

B. Acetaminophen

C. Duloxetine

D. Ketorolac

Q170. For pain management, which of the following medications are commonly utilized in Enhanced Recovery after Surgery (ERAS) protocols? (Select 3.)

A. Morphine

B. Fentanyl

C. Ketamine

D. Acetaminophen

E. Gabapentin

F. Lidocaine

Q171. What are the primary objectives of pain management strategies in Enhanced Recovery After Surgery (ERAS) protocols? (Select 3.)

A. Minimize opioid consumption

B. Promote early ambulation

C. Reduce postoperative nausea and vomiting

D. Enhance patient satisfaction

E. Expedite return of bowel function

F. Improve overall patient outcomes

Q172. What is the potential risk of using hypotensive techniques in anesthesia? (Select 3.)

A. Hyperthermia

B. Bradycardia

C. Hypertension

D. Tachypnea

E. Increased cardiac output

F. Elevated intracranial pressure

Q173. Which pharmacological agent is commonly used to induce controlled hypotension when using hypotensive anesthesia? (Select 3.)

A. Ephedrine

B. Phenylephrine

C. Nitroglycerin

D. Sodium nitroprusside

E. Clevidipine

F. Dexmedetomidine

Q174. During seizure prophylaxis in preeclampsia, the primary consideration for preventing magnesium toxicity is monitoring _____.

Q175. Fill in the blank: Intrathecal narcotic administration is associated with altered pain perception due to its effect on _____.

Q176. To prevent airborne transmission of pathogens in the operating room, which infection control measure is crucial for the anesthesia provider? (Select 3.)

A. Hand hygiene

B. Shoe covers

C. Gown

D. N95 respirator

E. Face shield

F. Hair cover

Q177. In the context of infection control, what is essential for the appropriate use of ultraviolet sanitizer in the anesthesia workplace? (Select 3.)

A. Frequency of handwashing

B. Distance from the UV source

C. Type of surgical gloves worn

D. Operating room temperature

E. Presence of laminar airflow

F. Compatibility with electronic equipment

Q178. Which infection control measure is important to prevent the spread of pathogens in the anesthesia workplace? (Select 2.)

A. Regular hand hygiene

B. Wearing personal protective equipment

C. Aseptic technique during procedures

D. Disinfecting equipment after each use

Q179. During surgery, which precaution is essential for preventing intraoperative fires?

A. High-flow oxygen delivery.

B. Increased use of flammable materials.

C. Prolonged use of electrocautery.

D. Minimal use of alcohol-based skin preparations.

Q180. What should be prioritized when choosing drapes and materials in the context of intraoperative fire safety?

A. Flame-retardant properties.

B. High oxygen concentration.

C. Ease of disposal.

D. Low cost.

Q181. For patients undergoing hepatobiliary surgery, which anesthetic consideration is particularly important?

A. Monitoring for nephrotoxicity

B. Avoiding neuromuscular blockade

C. Maintaining normothermia

D. Preventing hepatic ischemia-reperfusion injury

Q182. Which complication should be closely monitored due to its potential impact on patient outcomes during anesthesia for gastrointestinal tract procedures?

A. Renal insufficiency

B. Anaphylactic reactions

C. Hyperglycemia

D. Aspiration pneumonitis

Q183. Which complication is of particular concern due to its potential impact on metabolic homeostasis during anesthesia for endocrine organ procedures?

A. Hypertension

B. Hypothyroidism

C. Hypercalcemia

D. Hypoglycemia

Q184. Which intraoperative complication is of particular concern due to its potential impact on renal function, during anesthesia for renal/genitourinary procedures?

A. Hyperkalemia

B. Hyponatremia

C. Hypoglycemia

D. Acute tubular necrosis

Q185. Which complication may occur due to Trendelenburg positioning during anesthesia for gynecologic procedures?

A. Pulmonary embolism

B. Pneumothorax

C. Air embolism

D. Uterine atony

Q186. Which intraoperative complication is of primary concern, during anesthesia for peritoneal procedures such as hernia repair?

A. Hyperkalemia

B. Hepatic artery thrombosis

C. Pneumoperitoneum-induced hypercarbia

D. Delayed gastric emptying

Q187. Which complication is of primary concern due to its potential impact on surgical outcomes, during anesthesia for extrathoracic plastics and reconstructive procedures?

A. Hypothermia

B. Delayed emergence from anesthesia

C. Impaired wound healing

D. Electrolyte imbalance

Q188. Which nerve is most commonly at risk for injury during anesthesia for head extracranial otolaryngological procedures?

A. Facial nerve (CN VII)

B. Glossopharyngeal nerve (CN IX)

C. Trigeminal nerve (CN V)

D. Hypoglossal nerve (CN XII)

Q189. Which monitoring modality is essential for detecting changes in intracranial pressure, during anesthesia for intracranial decompression procedures such as burr holes or ventriculoperitoneal shunt placement?

A. Pulse oximetry

B. Capnography

C. Echocardiography

D. Invasive intracranial pressure monitoring

Q190. Which monitoring technique is essential for detecting cerebral perfusion changes and preventing cerebral ischemia during anesthesia for an intracranial space-occupying lesion?

A. Arterial blood gas analysis

B. Bispectral index monitoring

C. Transesophageal echocardiography

D. Intraoperative neurophysiologic monitoring

Q191. Which cardioplegia solution is commonly used to induce cardiac arrest during anesthesia for open cardiac procedures such as coronary artery bypass grafting (CABG)?

A. Ringer's lactate

B. Hartmann's solution

C. St. Thomas solution

D. Plasma-Lyte A

Q192. Which is the primary hemodynamic goal to optimize cardiac output and minimize myocardial injury during transcatheter aortic valve replacement (TAVR/TAVI)?

A. Decrease systemic vascular resistance

B. Increase preload

C. Maintain sinus rhythm

D. Prevent aortic regurgitation

Q193. Which intervention is crucial to prevent device dislodgement and ensure proper lead placement during anesthesia for pacemaker implantation?

A. Maintaining stable anesthesia depth

B. Monitoring for signs of pneumothorax

C. Administering antiarrhythmic medications

D. Avoiding neuromuscular blockade reversal

Q194. Which intervention is critical to prevent device-related complications, during anesthesia for a patient with an intraarterial balloon pump?

A. Monitoring for signs of pulmonary embolism

B. Maintaining adequate anticoagulation levels

C. Ensuring proper positioning of the arterial catheter

D. Administering vasopressors to maintain perfusion

Q195. Which complication should be carefully monitored due to its association with diaphragmatic manipulation, during anesthesia for a patient undergoing diaphragmatic surgery?

A. Pneumothorax

B. Pulmonary embolism

C. Acute respiratory distress syndrome (ARDS)

D. Phrenic nerve injury

Q196. Which complication should be anticipated due to airway manipulation and potential trauma, during anesthesia for a bronchoscopy procedure?

A. Hypotension

B. Bradycardia

C. Hypoxemia

D. Hyperthermia

Q197. Which complications should the nurse anesthetist be vigilant for during anesthesia for esophageal surgery? (Select 2)

A. Aspiration pneumonitis

B. Esophageal perforation

C. Mediastinitis

D. Vocal cord paralysis

Q198. Which complications should the nurse anesthetist be vigilant for, during anesthesia for lung surgery? (Select 2)

A. Bronchopleural fistula

B. Acute respiratory distress syndrome (ARDS)

C. Pneumothorax

D. Aspiration pneumonia

Q199. Which complications should the nurse anesthetist be vigilant for, during anesthesia for mediastinal surgery? (Select 2)

A. Tracheal compression

B. Air embolism

C. Esophageal perforation

D. Horner's syndrome

Q200. Which complications should the nurse anesthetist be vigilant for, during anesthesia for procedures involving the neck? (Select 2)

A. Airway edema

B. Vocal cord paralysis

C. Tracheal stenosis

D. Esophageal perforation

Q201. Which complications should be carefully monitored during anesthesia for neck lymph node biopsies? (Select 2)

A. Airway obstruction

B. Bleeding

C. Nerve injury

D. Respiratory depression

Q202. What is a critical consideration for preventing nerve injury during anesthesia for parathyroid/thyroid surgeries? (Select 2)

A. Avoiding hypotension

B. Monitoring recurrent laryngeal nerve integrity

C. Administering high-dose opioids

D. Maintaining deep levels of anesthesia

Q203. What is a crucial consideration to prevent complications during neuroskeletal surgeries? (Select2)

A. Monitoring for hypoglycemia

B. Administering muscle relaxants

C. Avoiding excessive head movement

D. Increasing intraoperative fluids

Q204. Which anesthesia consideration is essential to prevent complications during arthroscopic procedures? (Select 2)

A. Administering local anesthesia only

B. Monitoring for compartment syndrome

C. Maintaining normothermia

D. Minimizing intraoperative fluid administration

Q205. Which anesthesia consideration is essential to minimize postoperative complications during anal/rectal procedures? (Select 2)

A. Use of general anesthesia only

B. Continuous monitoring of bowel motility

C. Adequate pain control for patient comfort

D. Limiting preoperative fasting to minimize fluid loss

Q206. Which factor influences the choice between open and endovascular procedures during vascular surgery? (Select 2)

A. Patient age and gender

B. Complexity of the lesion and anatomy

C. Availability of operating room equipment

D. Surgeon's preference and experience

Q207. Which factors are crucial for managing occlusive disease and ensuring appropriate vascular access during anesthesia for extremity procedures? (Select 2)

A. Preoperative imaging and patient positioning

B. Maintenance of adequate perfusion and arterial cannulation

C. Administration of regional anesthesia and monitoring of peripheral pulses

D. Utilization of vasoactive medications and postoperative wound care

Q208. Which interventions are essential to minimize the risk of clot formation in anesthesia for thromboembolic prevention? (Select 2)

A. Administration of anticoagulant medications and vigilant monitoring for signs of bleeding

B. Utilization of pneumatic compression devices and maintaining normothermia

C. Avoidance of regional anesthesia techniques and aggressive fluid resuscitation

D. Application of prophylactic antibiotics and strict control of intraoperative blood pressure

Q209. Which interventions are crucial to mitigate the risk of bleeding in the surgical management of portal hypertension? (Select 2)

A. Selective portal vein embolization and transjugular intrahepatic portosystemic shunt (TIPS)

B. Splenectomy and devascularization procedures

C. Prophylactic administration of vasopressors and careful hemodynamic monitoring

D. Placement of a mesocaval shunt and hepatic artery ligation

Q210. Which factors contribute to the risk of intra-abdominal insufflation-related complications during robotic/laparoscopic surgery? (Select 2)

A. Increased intra-abdominal pressure and impaired venous return

B. Reduced intra-abdominal pressure and enhanced tissue perfusion

C. Enhanced venous return and decreased respiratory compromise

D. Decreased intra-abdominal pressure and improved cardiac output

Q211. Regarding pediatric airway anatomy, which of the following statements is true? (Select 3)

A. The epiglottis is relatively larger and U-shaped in infants.

B. The cricoid cartilage is the narrowest part of the pediatric airway.

C. The trachea is shorter and more flexible in children compared to adults.

D. The larynx is positioned higher in the neck in pediatric patients.

E. The pediatric glottis is narrower and more anterior than in adults.

F. The tongue is proportionally smaller in infants compared to adults.

Q212. Which physiological differences in pediatric patients contribute to the increased risk of hypothermia? (Select 3)

A. Higher surface area-to-volume ratio

B. Reduced subcutaneous fat insulation

C. Limited shivering response

D. Immature thermoregulatory mechanisms

E. Increased metabolic rate

F. Decreased ability to vasoconstrict

Q213. Which of the following are typical physiological characteristics of premature neonates? (Select 3)

A. Decreased alveolar surface area

B. Immature thermoregulation

C. Underdeveloped pulmonary surfactant production

D. Limited glycogen stores

E. Increased risk of hypoglycemia

F. Immature liver function

Q214. Which of the following anatomical features distinguish the airway of premature neonates from that of term neonates? (Select 3)

A. Larger diameter trachea

B. More developed cartilaginous structures

C. Presence of bronchial cartilage rings

D. Smaller number of alveoli

E. Increased airway resistance

F. Thinner and less compliant chest wall

Q215. During embryonic development, which congenital abnormalities are characterized by a failure of the neural tube to close? (Select 3)

A. Spina bifida

B. Congenital diaphragmatic hernia

C. Esophageal atresia

D. Tracheoesophageal fistula

E. Hirschsprung's disease

F. Cleft lip and palate

Q216. In pediatric patients, which opioid analgesics are commonly used due to its short duration of action and minimal accumulation? (Select 3)

A. Morphine

B. Fentanyl

C. Hydromorphone

D. Oxycodone

E. Methadone

F. Codeine

Q217. What techniques involve injecting a local anesthetic around a nerve trunk and are used for pediatric peripheral nerve blocks to provide regional anesthesia? (Select 3)

A. Caudal block

B. Intercostal nerve block

C. Brachial plexus block

D. Fascia iliaca compartment block

E. Popliteal nerve block

F. Axillary nerve block

Q218. What complications are associated with pediatric airway management using a laryngeal mask airway (LMA)? (Select 3)

A. Aspiration

B. Laryngospasm

C. Esophageal intubation

D. Oropharyngeal trauma

E. Hypoxemia

F. Bronchospasm

Q219. What anatomical changes occur during pregnancy that contribute to an increased risk of aspiration during anesthesia? (Select 3)

A. Decreased gastric emptying

B. Increased lower esophageal sphincter tone

C. Elevated diaphragm position

D. Decreased intra-abdominal pressure

E. Increased airway diameter

F. Enhanced cough reflex

Q220. Which of the following medications are typically administered to prevent preterm labor and fetal distress during tocolysis? (Select 3)

A. Ritodrine

B. Fentanyl

C. Ephedrine

D. Ketorolac

E. Succinylcholine

F. Rocuronium

Q221. In patients desiring mobility, what anesthesia procedure is recommended for labor analgesia? (Select 3)

A. Continuous epidural analgesia

B. Intravenous patient-controlled analgesia (PCA)

C. Intermittent bolus epidural analgesia

D. Combined spinal-epidural analgesia

E. Transcutaneous electrical nerve stimulation (TENS)

F. Pudendal nerve block

Q222. During cesarean delivery, which anesthesia considerations are crucial for managing a high-risk parturient with a history of placenta accreta? (Select 3)

A. Blood product availability

B. Obstetric hemorrhage protocol

C. Rapid access to interventional radiology

D. Preoperative multidisciplinary planning

E. Fetal monitoring expertise

F. Uterine artery embolization readiness

Q223. For a parturient with a history of placenta previa, which anesthesia techniques are suitable for nonobstetric surgery? (Select 3)

A. Regional anesthesia to minimize bleeding risk

B. General anesthesia with rapid sequence induction

C. Preoperative administration of tocolytic agents

D. Continuous fetal heart rate monitoring during surgery

E. Strict avoidance of uterine contractions intraoperatively

F. Preoperative evaluation for fetal lung maturity

Q224. In the management of a parturient with suspected amniotic fluid embolism (AFE), which interventions are crucial? (Select 3)

A. Immediate initiation of cardiopulmonary resuscitation (CPR)

B. Administration of vasopressors to maintain blood pressure

C. Emergent cesarean delivery if fetal distress is present

D. Prompt initiation of massive transfusion protocol

E. Rapid institution of advanced airway management

F. Administration of intravenous calcium to counter hypocalcemia

Q225. Which pharmacologic agent is commonly used to augment uterine contraction in the management of postpartum hemorrhage? (Select 3)

A. Oxytocin

B. Nitroglycerin

C. Ephedrine

D. Norepinephrine

E. Methylergonovine

F. Misoprostol

Q226. What physiological changes in the elderly patients increases the risk of drug accumulation and prolonged effects? (Select 3)

A. Increased hepatic blood flow

B. Decreased renal function

C. Enhanced gastrointestinal motility

D. Augmented drug metabolism

E. Elevated lean body mass

F. Reduced volume of distribution

Q227. Due to alterations in pharmacokinetics and pharmacodynamics, elderly patients often exhibit _____ sensitivity to opioids.

Q228. Adjusting the _____ is crucial to prevent systemic toxicity and achieve adequate anesthesia in geriatric patients during regional anesthesia.

Q229. Vigilant monitoring and early recognition of signs of _____ are essential for mitigating the risk of postoperative cognitive dysfunction in geriatric patients.

Q230. Alterations in _____ during anesthesia can lead to increased risk of airway obstruction and difficult mask ventilation in obese patients.

Q231. Because of alterations in adipose tissue distribution and metabolism in obese patients, the volume of distribution of lipophilic drugs such as _____ may be altered.

Q232. Utilizing the _____ technique is the preferred airway management approach to facilitate intubation and minimize the risk of complications in obese patients during bariatric anesthesia.

Q233. To prevent postoperative respiratory compromise and hypoxemia, vigilance for _____ is crucial in managing complications of obesity during anesthesia.

Q234. Caution is warranted during anesthesia due to the potential for _____, which may require adjustments in opioid dosing in patients receiving medication-assisted therapy (MAT) for substance use disorder.

Q235. During acute intoxication, patients with substance use disorder are at risk of experiencing _____ interactions with anesthetics, necessitating careful drug selection and titration.

Q236. A multimodal approach, combining _____ medications with non-pharmacologic interventions, is necessary for effective pain management in patients with substance use disorder.

Q237. Vigilant monitoring for _____, such as respiratory depression and hemodynamic instability, is required during the management of substance use disorder patients undergoing anesthesia.

Q238. Anesthetic agents must be chosen carefully to reduce _____ and maintain adequate immune function in immune-compromised and oncology patients.

Q239. Meticulous attention to aseptic technique during _____ is crucial to prevent infections and complications in immune-compromised and oncology patients.

Q240. Close monitoring of vital signs and _____ is essential for promptly addressing any adverse events or complications in managing anesthesia for immune-compromised and oncology patients.

Test Answer Key

Q1.

Answer: A

Explanation: Heart rate is the primary determinant of myocardial oxygen consumption because it directly influences oxygen demand. This action makes it a crucial factor during anesthesia management.

Q2.

Answer: A

Explanation: Diastolic blood pressure correlates strongly with coronary perfusion pressure during CPR and becomes crucial for coronary artery perfusion.

Q3.

Answer: C

Explanation: Increased airway resistance leads to reduced expiratory flow rates, which reflects difficulty in moving air out of the lungs.

Q4.

Answer: A

Explanation: Respiratory rate is crucial for gas exchange in the lungs. It determines the frequency of alveolar ventilation.

Q5.

Answer: C

Explanation: GABA acts as the primary inhibitory neurotransmitter in the central nervous system. It regulates neuronal excitability and maintains balance.

Q6.

Answer: A

Explanation: The cerebellum is the brain region most likely to result in deficits, and it plays a crucial role in coordinating voluntary movements and maintaining balance. This role makes it essential for motor control.

Q7.

Answer: B

Explanation: Tendons connect muscles to bones, transmitting forces generated by muscle contractions. This transmission produces movement or stabilizes joints in the musculoskeletal system.

Q8.

Answer: B

Explanation: Glucagon stimulates glycogenolysis in the liver, which releases glucose into the bloodstream. Its purpose is to increase blood glucose levels, counteracting hypoglycemia.

Q9.

Answer: B

Explanation: During the process of urine formation, renal tubules reabsorb water and essential nutrients from the filtrate. It returns them to the bloodstream.

Q10.

Answer: C

Explanation: Erythropoietin is produced by the kidneys and stimulates red blood cell production in response to low oxygen levels in the blood.

Q11.

Answer: C

Explanation: Gastrin stimulates the secretion of hydrochloric acid and pepsinogen, which aids in digestion.

Q12.

Answer: B

Explanation: B cells produce antibodies as part of the humoral immune response. They play a key role in defense against pathogens.

Q13.

Answer: B and C

Explanation: Troponin I and myoglobin are specific markers for myocardial injury. These both aid in the diagnosis of ischemic heart disease.

Q14.

Answer: A and C

Explanation: Aortic and mitral regurgitation both cause diastolic murmurs and widened pulse pressure due to backflow into the left ventricle during diastole.

Q15.

Answer: A and B

Explanation: Asthma and chronic bronchitis both involve reversible airflow limitation and airway inflammation, which distinguishes them from emphysema and bronchiectasis.

Q16.

Answer: A and B

Explanation: Both Parkinson's and Alzheimer's diseases involve Lewy bodies and impair both motor and cognitive functions.

Q17.

Answer: A and D

Explanation: Hyperkalemia and hyperthermia increases the risk of malignant hyperthermia during anesthesia induction.

Q18.

Answer: B and D

Explanation: Parathyroid hormone (PTH) increases blood calcium levels through mechanisms such as promoting calcium release from bones. Whereas calcitonin decreases them by promoting bone deposition.

Q19.

Answer: B and C

Explanation: Both hepatitis B and hepatitis C are viral infections that predominantly target the liver. These infections lead to inflammation and potential long-term complications.

Q20.

Answer: A and B

Explanation: Both IgA nephropathy and nephrotic syndrome show problems in the kidneys that cause blood in urine, protein in urine, and high blood pressure.

Q21.

Answer: A and B

Explanation: Thalassemia and sickle cell anemia both exhibit target cells and increased hemoglobin F levels.

Q22.

Answer: A and D

Explanation: Gastroesophageal reflux disease (GERD) and Hiatal hernia both exhibit backward flow of stomach acid and regurgitation of food.

Q23.

Answer: A and B

Explanation: HIV/AIDS is a medical condition that weakens the immune system, leading to susceptibility to opportunistic infections like tuberculosis.

Q24.

Answer: A and D

Explanation: Characteristic features of cancer cells involve uncontrolled cell growth and restored cell cycle regulation, which leads to tumor formation.

Q25.

Answer: E, F, and D

Explanation: Halothane, xenon, and isoflurane have higher blood/gas partition coefficients, which leads to slower induction and recovery compared to other inhalation anesthetics.

Q26.

Answer: A, B, and C

Explanation: Pancuronium, vecuronium, and rocuronium are nondepolarizing neuromuscular blocking agents, which competitively antagonize acetylcholine at the nicotinic receptor.

Q27.

Answer: A, D, and E

Explanation: Bupivacaine, ropivacaine, and tetracaine are long-acting local anesthetics that block sodium channels, making them suitable for spinal anesthesia.

Q28.

Answer: B, C, and F

Explanation: Lipid emulsion therapy, intravenous bicarbonate, and intravenous dantrolene are utilized to manage LAST by sequestering lipid-soluble drugs and buffering metabolic acidosis, respectively.

Q29.

Answer: B, C, and D

Explanation: Clonidine, dexmedetomidine, and dexamethasone are commonly used as adjuvants in regional anesthesia to prolong sensory blockade and analgesia.

Q30.

Answer: A, B, and C

Explanation: Atropine and glycopyrrolate are anticholinergics, while neostigmine is a cholinergic agonist, often used to reverse neuromuscular blockade and increase gastrointestinal motility in anesthesia practice.

Q31.

Answer: A, B, and D

Explanation: Acetaminophen, NSAIDs, and gabapentin are non-opioid analgesics frequently used in anesthesia practice for pain management without the risks associated with opioid medications.

Q32.

Answer: A, B, and D

Explanation: To improve bronchial airflow and facilitate ventilation during anesthesia, bronchodilators like albuterol, ipratropium, and formoterol are frequently administered.

Q33.

Answers: A, D, and E

Explanation: Prostaglandins exert various effects including vasodilation, uterine contraction, and inhibition of platelet aggregation. They make them useful in several clinical contexts such as managing hypertension and inducing labor.

Q34.

Answers: A, B, and D

Explanation: Histamine receptor antagonists block the action of histamine which leads to decreased gastric acid secretion, prevention of gastric ulcers, and relief of allergic symptoms.

Q35.

Answers: A, B, and C

Explanation: Insulin stimulates glycogen synthesis, promotes glucose uptake by cells, and inhibits hepatic glucose production. Thereby, it reduces blood glucose levels and promotes energy storage.

Q36.

Answers: A, B, and C

Explanation: Hypoglycemic medications can work by promoting insulin release from pancreatic beta cells, enhancing insulin sensitivity in peripheral tissues, and inhibiting hepatic glucose production which ultimately leads to reduced blood glucose levels.

Q37.

Answer: Molarity

Explanation: Molarity (M) is used in chemistry to quantify the concentration of a solution. It is a measure of concentration defined as the number of moles of solute dissolved per liter of solution.

Q38.

Answer: water

Explanation: In a neutralization reaction between an acid and a base HCl (acid) reacts with NaOH (base) to produce NaCl (salt) and water.

Q39.

Answer: oxidation

Explanation: During cellular respiration, glucose is oxidized which releases energy that is used to produce ATP along with carbon dioxide and water as byproducts.

Q40.

Answer: glycolysis

Explanation: Glucose undergoes glycolysis to produce ATP energy and pyruvate which involves a series of enzymatic reactions. Then it enters the citric acid cycle where further oxidation occurs which leads to the production of additional ATP and carbon dioxide.

Q41.

Answer: receptor

Explanation: Signal transduction begins with the binding of a ligand to a receptor on the cell membrane which triggers intracellular signaling pathways and cellular responses.

Q42.

Answer: antagonists

Explanation: By binding to receptors without activating them, antagonists block the action of agonists and prevent their response.

Q43.

Answer: meter

Explanation: The meter, symbolized by "m", is defined as the distance traveled by light in a vacuum in 1/299,792,458 of a second. It is the fundamental unit of length in the SI system.

Q44.

Answer: inversely

Explanation: Boyle's law states that the pressure of a gas is inversely proportional to its volume at a constant temperature, i.e. as volume increases, pressure decreases, and vice versa.

Q45.

Answer: directly

Explanation: Fick's law of diffusion states that the rate of diffusion of a gas across a membrane is directly proportional to the surface area and the concentration gradient i.e. as the surface area or concentration gradient increases, the diffusion rate increases.

Q46.

Answer: directly

Explanation: According to Poiseuille's law, the flow rate of a fluid through a cylindrical tube is directly proportional to the pressure gradient and the fourth power of the radius.

Q47.

Answer: grounded

Explanation: By providing a path for current to safely dissipate into the ground, proper grounding of electrical circuits helps to prevent electrical shock which reduces the risk of electric shock to individuals.

Q48.

Answer: volume

Explanation: This formula helps in determining the volume of medication needed based on its concentration, desired dose, and patient's weight which ensures accurate drug administration.

Q49.

Answer: B.

Explanation: Due to their portability and consistent pressure delivery, cylinder gases stored under high pressure are commonly used as a gas source for anesthesia delivery systems.

Q50.

Answer: C.

Explanation: Regulators ensure patient safety and equipment functionality. They are responsible for controlling the pressure of gas from high-pressure cylinders to levels suitable for anesthesia delivery systems.

Q51.

Answer: B.

Explanation: Flowmeters regulate gas flow by controlling the size of the orifice. During anesthesia administration, they allow precise adjustment of gas delivery rates.

Q52.

Answer: B.

Explanation: Vaporizers ensure precise delivery of the desired concentration to the patient during anesthesia by converting liquid anesthetic agents into a vaporized form.

Q53.

Answer: C.

Explanation: During anesthesia induction and maintenance, proportioning systems precisely mix oxygen and volatile anesthetic agents in the desired concentrations for delivery to the patient.

Q54.

Answer: D.

Explanation: Pressure failure safety devices are crucial components of anesthetic delivery systems. They prevent the administration of anesthetic gases in case of a loss of gas pressure and ensure patient safety during anesthesia.

Q55.

Answer: C

Explanation: For safe and effective anesthesia delivery, the proportioning system controls the mix of gases to maintain the desired concentration.

Q56.

Answer: D.

Explanation: Dual control in ventilators enhances patient safety during mechanical ventilation. This feature adjusts both pressure and volume to maintain consistent tidal volumes despite variations in lung compliance or airway resistance.

Q57.

Answer: A.

Explanation: Soda lime reacts with exhaled carbon dioxide and converts it into calcium carbonate and water, thus preventing rebreathing of carbon dioxide during anesthesia. It is a widely used carbon dioxide absorbent in anesthesia machines.

Q58.

Answer: B.

Explanation: In a circle anesthesia system, the reservoir bag acts as a visual indicator of patient ventilation. It expands during inspiration and collapse during expiration which allows the anesthetist to monitor the patient's respiratory status.

Q59.

Answer: B.

Explanation: Non-rebreathing circuits reduce the risk of carbon dioxide buildup, improve patient safety and prevent the rebreathing of exhaled gases.

Q60.

Answer: B.

Explanation: Pneumatic and electronic alarm devices are crucial in anesthesia to provide audible and visual alerts for abnormal conditions which enhances patient safety.

Q61.

Answer A and B.

Explanation: Face masks in anesthesia ensure efficient ventilation and prevent air leakage by providing a tight seal over the patient's nose and mouth, enabling for the delivery of high concentrations of oxygen.

Q62.

Answer A and B.

Explanation: A laryngoscope facilitates successful intubation by providing direct visualization of the vocal cords, aiding in proper placement of the endotracheal tube into the trachea.

Q63.

Answer A and C.

Explanation: When using a flexible fiberoptic bronchoscope for intubation, it is necessary to navigate through anatomical structures effectively and to use of topical anesthesia to reduce patient discomfort.

Q64.

Answer: B and D.

Explanation: To prevent mucosal damage and ensure an effective seal against aspiration, endotracheal tube cuffs should maintain a high volume and low pressure.

Q65.

Answer: A and C.

Explanation: It is important to consider the size of the distal cuff for sealing and placement of the bronchial lumen for lung isolation when selecting a double-lumen endobronchial tube.

Q66.

Answer: A and C.

Explanation: Consider the blocker size for proper occlusion and positioning when selecting a bronchial blocker for lung isolation.

Q67.

Answer: B and C.

Explanation: Accommodating the patient's anatomy during selection involves considering the diameter for appropriate fit and flexibility.

Q68.

Answer: A and C.

Explanation: It is crucial to consider the size for appropriate fit and flexibility to accommodate nasal anatomy comfortably during proper selection.

Q69.

Answer: A and C.

Explanation: Consider the inner diameter for adequate airflow and the presence of a cuff for sealing the airway when selecting a tracheostomy tube.

Q70.

Answer: A and C.

Explanation: Proper placement of the LMA include the assessment of bilateral chest rise and symmetrical chest movement to ensure adequate ventilation.

Q71.

Answer: B and D.

Explanation: It is essential to ensure adequate ventilation and verify correct placement with capnography to detect the presence of exhaled CO_2 levels before advancing the endotracheal tube.

Q72.

Answer: A and B.

Explanation: By regulating airflow and delivering oxygen directly to the surgical field, jet ventilation offers advantages such as reduced risk of barotrauma and enhanced surgical exposure.

Q73.

Answer: A, C, E.

Explanation: Intubating stylets contribute to improved maneuverability, aiding in endotracheal tube placement and facilitating passage through anatomical obstructions, thus reducing the risk of soft tissue injury in difficult airway scenarios.

Q74.

Answer: A, B, C.

Explanation: Cricothyrotomy is indicated when endotracheal intubation fails, severe upper airway obstruction occurs, or urgent airway access is required to prevent hypoxia or death in emergency airway management.

Q75.

Answer: A, B, C.

Explanation: Intubation aids such as airway exchange catheters, endotracheal tube introducers, and gum elastic bougies provide additional guidance or alternative methods for tube placement, facilitating tracheal intubation in patients with challenging airways.

Q76.

Answer: C, D, F.

Explanation: The EEG, NIRS, and SSEP monitor provides valuable information during anesthesia by assessing evoked potentials in response to various stimuli, allowing for the monitoring of central nervous system function.

Q77.

Answer: C, F, D.

Explanation: To directly measure intracranial pressure, cardiac output, and tissue oxygenation in neurosurgical patients, the intracranial pressure (ICP) monitor, pulse contour cardiac output (PiCCO) monitor, and transcutaneous oxygen saturation monitor are utilized.

Q78.

Answer: B, E, F.

Explanation: The Bispectral Index (BIS) monitor is essential for monitoring anesthesia depth and assessing cerebral function by analyzing EEG activity. Additionally, the Intracranial pressure (ICP) monitor measures skull pressure, indicating conditions such as trauma, while Near-infrared spectroscopy (NIRS) monitors cerebral oxygenation during surgery.

Q79.

Answer: A, D, C.

Explanation: Assessing neuromuscular blockade involves using the Train-of-four (TOF) monitor and peripheral nerve stimulator, which stimulates peripheral nerves and measures muscle response. Additionally, the Bispectral Index (BIS) monitor, primarily used for assessing cerebral function, also guides the titration of anesthetic drugs during surgery.

Q80.

Answer: A, C, F.

Explanation: Lead I, Lead II, and Lead III are typically included in a standard 3-lead ECG, providing information on different aspects of cardiac electrical activity and axis.

Q81.

Answer: B, C, and D.

Explanation: During the anesthesia, continuous arterial pressure monitoring is typically achieved using an arterial line, providing real-time blood pressure measurements essential for hemodynamic management.

Q82.

Answer: B, D, and F.

Explanation: For accurate and reliable measurements, noninvasive blood pressure monitoring in anesthetized patients often involves the use of a Doppler ultrasound, oscillometric blood pressure cuff, or continuous cardiac output monitor.

Q83.

Answers: B, C, F

Explanation: In this scenario, the nurse anesthetist's error involves breaching the duty of care and may lead to harm. The legal principles at play include informed consent, emphasizing the importance of clear communication with patients, and disclosure of errors/injuries, highlighting the obligation to inform patients about mistakes for ethical and legal reasons.

Q84.

Answer: C, D, and E.

Explanation: For accurate assessment of intravascular volume status, central venous pressure monitoring is typically performed using a central venous catheter, arterial line transducer, or Doppler ultrasound.

Q85.

Answer: D, E, and C.

Explanation: Transesophageal echocardiography can provide information about pulmonary artery pressure. Pulmonary artery pressure and SvO2 are typically measured using a pulmonary artery catheter equipped with a fiber optic sensor or a Swan-Ganz catheter.

Q86.

Answer: C, D, and F.

Explanation: In real-time, arterial, line waveform analysis, pulmonary artery catheterization (PAC), and impedance cardiography are monitoring techniques used to assess various hemodynamic parameters.

Q87.

Answer: Transesophageal

Explanation: Transesophageal echocardiography (TEE) allows clinicians to visualize cardiac anatomy and function with high resolution. It is an essential intraoperative monitoring tool.

Q88.

Answer: carbon dioxide (CO_2)

Explanation: In exhaled breath, capnography measures the concentration of carbon dioxide. It offers valuable insights into respiratory status and aids in promptly identifying respiratory complications.

Q89.

Answer: end-tidal carbon dioxide (EtCO2)

Explanation: Monitoring end-tidal carbon dioxide levels helps identify issues such as airway obstruction or hypoventilation, enhances patient safety during anesthesia, and allows for continuous assessment of ventilation adequacy.

Q90.

Answer: Electrical

Explanation: To assess the degree of neuromuscular blockade, the peripheral nerve stimulator delivers electrical impulses. It helps anesthesia providers determine the need for reversal agents and monitor patient recovery from muscle relaxation.

Q91.

Answer: Skin

Explanation: During anesthesia, skin temperature probes are frequently utilized for continuous monitoring. It aids in the prevention of hypothermia or hyperthermia and provides valuable information about the patient's thermal status.

Q92.

Answer: hypothermia

Explanation: In preventing hypothermia, fluid/blood warmers play a crucial role, particularly in patients undergoing surgery where significant fluid replacement is required. It reduces the risk of adverse outcomes associated with perioperative hypothermia.

Q93.

Answer: hypothermia

Explanation: Forced air warming devices are commonly used intraoperatively to prevent hypothermia and maintain normothermia in surgical patients, which is associated with adverse outcomes such as increased bleeding, surgical site infections, and delayed recovery.

Q94.

Answer: expeditiously

Explanation: Rapid infusers are utilized intraoperatively to deliver large volumes of fluids and blood products expeditiously. It aids in the swift replenishment of intravascular volume, particularly in situations requiring urgent fluid resuscitation.

Q95.

Answer: Guidance

Explanation: Ultrasound provides real-time imaging, during anesthesia procedures, it aids in the precise localization of structures. Thereby it may improve procedural accuracy and patient safety.

Q96.

Answer: interventional pain management or cardiac catheterization

Explanation: Fluoroscopy is a real-time imaging technique that uses X-rays to visualize structures within the body, aiding in procedures such as interventional pain management or cardiac catheterization.

Q97.

Answer A.

Explanation: Respecting patient's values and preferences, autonomy emphasizes a patient's right to make decisions about their own care.

Q98.

Answer C.

Explanation: When considering beneficence in anesthesia practice, providing optimal pain management promotes the patient's well-being.

Q99.

Answer: A.

Explanation: In research ethics, autonomy emphasizes the requirement to obtain voluntary, informed consent from participants.

Q100.

Answer: B.

Explanation: Beneficence obliges researchers to seek the well-being of research participants by ensuring that the benefits of the study outweigh potential harms and by maximizing the benefits while minimizing risks.

Q101.

Answer A and D.

Explanation: In the context of Advance Healthcare Directives, autonomy protection ensures that an anesthetist respects a patient's previously stated wishes about end-of-life care. Veracity underscores the obligation to truthfully inform patients about their care.

Q102.

Answer B and D.

Explanation: A durable power of attorney for healthcare designates a healthcare proxy, while a POLST form guides specific medical interventions based on patient preferences. Both are crucial in honoring Advance Healthcare Directives.

Q103.

Answer: C and D.

Explanation: In the context of legal considerations, a family member's opinion and detailed explanation of risks and benefits is essential for obtaining valid informed consent before administering anesthesia.

Q104.

Answer: A and D.

Explanation: When addressing legal aspects of informed consent, the anesthesia provider's notes and witnessed patient refusal form are crucial for legal protection and demonstrating the informed consent process.

Q105.

Answers: B, C, F

Explanation: In this scenario, the nurse anesthetist's error involves breaching the duty of care and may lead to harm. The legal principles at play include informed consent, emphasizing the importance of clear communication with patients, and disclosure of errors/injuries, highlighting the obligation to inform patients about mistakes for ethical and legal reasons.

Q106.

Answers: B, E, F

Explanation: In the context of legal doctrines related to anesthesia practice, Informed consent mandates providing comprehensive information to the patient, assuring their understanding. Assumption of risk and Good Samaritan laws are legal considerations.

Q107.

Answer A, C, F.

Explanation: In this case, the legal concepts of res ipsa loquitur, strict liability, and comparative negligence are most relevant. Res ipsa loquitur is relevant when an injury would not occur in the absence of negligence. Strict liability holds parties responsible regardless of fault, and comparative negligence compares the plaintiff's negligence with the defendant's.

Q108.

Answers: A, F

Explanation: In the context of legal issues and scope of practice, Nurse Anesthetists are authorized to administer blood transfusions and provide postoperative pain management within their scope of practice. These activities align with their role in perioperative care.

Q109.

Answer: State Nurse Practice Act

Explanation: The State Nurse Practice Act defines the legal scope of practice for nurse anesthetists. It ensures adherence to defined roles and responsibilities to provide safe and competent care.

Q110.

Answer: American Association of Nurse Anesthetists (AANA)

Explanation: For maintaining professional standards in nurse anesthesia practice, adherence to AANA guidelines is crucial which ensures ethical conduct and legal compliance for optimal patient outcomes.

Q111.

Answer: CPT (Current Procedural Terminology) codes.

Explanation: It is essential to include the CPT codes in anesthesia procedures. It ensures transparent representation of the procedures performed, adheres to legal standards, and facilitates proper reimbursement.

Q112.

Answer: decreased

Explanation: To ensure appropriate reimbursement for anesthesia services, proper documentation of medical necessity is essential. Failure to meet legal billing requirements may result in decreased reimbursement rates and legal ramifications for the provider.

Q113.

Answer: D.

Explanation: For patient safety, recognizing signs of substance abuse in a colleague is crucial. Seeking guidance from a professional support program ensures a confidential and supportive approach to addressing the issue.

Q114.

Answer: C.

Explanation: Among anesthesia providers, offering confidential counseling services while addressing substance abuse fosters a supportive environment. It promotes safety, wellness, and early intervention for substance abuse issues.

Q115.

Answer B.

Explanation: To ensure patient safety in the administration of anesthesia, thorough knowledge of allergies and sensitivities is crucial.

Q116.

Answer A.

Explanation: To reduce the risk of medication errors and promote a collaborative approach to patient care, double-checking drug labels with a colleague is a key safety measure.

Q117.

Answer C and D.

Explanation: Immediate action involves notifying the supervisor to address the situation promptly and relieving the impaired provider to ensure optimal patient care. As recognizing impaired provider performance is crucial for patient safety.

Q118.

Answer A and D.

Explanation: To ensure wellness and safety, an effective peer monitoring system involves regular assessments of cognitive and psychomotor skills, fostering a culture of mutual support. Ignoring subtle changes in behavior can compromise patient safety, emphasizing the importance of vigilant monitoring.

Q119.

Answer B and D.

Explanation: For stress reduction and enhancing mental well-being among healthcare professionals, regular mindfulness meditation and participation in peer assistance workshops are proven strategies.

Q120.

Answer B and D.

Explanation: To ensure accountability and maintain a safe practice environment, peer assistance programs contribute to safety and wellness by offering support for substance abuse issues and conducting surprise evaluations.

Q121.

Answer: C, D, F.

Explanation: When assessing a patient with severe aortic stenosis preoperatively, careful preoperative assessment and management are essential to optimize outcomes, as severe aortic stenosis poses risks of tachycardia, hypotension, and increased afterload.

Q122.

Answer: A, B, D.

Explanation: In COPD patients, optimizing bronchodilation, promoting smoking cessation, and using incentive spirometry can help reduce perioperative complications, ensuring better outcomes.

Q123.

Answer: A, B, D

Explanation: For assessing intravascular volume status in critically ill patients, central venous pressure (CVP), urine output, and pulmonary artery wedge pressure (PAWP) are considered valuable indicators.

Q124.

Answer: B, C, E

Explanation: During fluid therapy in patients with septic shock, albumin, crystalloid, and plasma expander solutions are effective in improving outcomes as suggested by studies. These options should be considered based on individual patient characteristics and clinical context.

Q125.

Answers: B, E, F.

Explanation: Fluid management in bloodless medicine involves crystalloid support, blood salvage devices for reinfusion, and hemodilution techniques to optimize patient outcomes.

Q126.

Answers: C, D, F.

Explanation: Preoperative iron supplementation improves hemoglobin levels, intraoperative cell salvage reduces blood loss, and vasopressors maintain hemodynamic stability, collectively minimizing the need for allogeneic blood transfusions in bloodless medicine.

Q127.

Answer: hemodynamic parameters

Explanation: Goal-directed fluid management aims to optimize cardiac output, commonly monitored through hemodynamic parameters like stroke volume and heart rate, ensuring efficient tissue perfusion.

Q128.

Answer: stroke volume variation

Explanation: Stroke volume variation is a dynamic parameter used in goal-directed fluid management to assess fluid responsiveness and guide fluid administration to optimize cardiac output.

Q129.

Answer: Fluid volume assessment

Explanation: Continuous fluid volume assessment is crucial during massive transfusion to avoid complications such as fluid overload or hypovolemia, ensuring optimal patient outcomes.

Q130.

Answer C.

Explanation: To evaluate hemostasis and guide transfusion decisions, platelet count is crucial. Thromboelastography complements this by providing dynamic insights into clot formation and strength.

Q131.

Answer A.

Explanation: Thromboelastography (TEG) by offering real-time information on clot formation and strength, assesses platelet function and the entire coagulation cascade. This aids in tailoring coagulation support for surgical patients.

Q132.

Answer: D.

Explanation: During anesthetic management, patients with a history of myotonic dystrophy may benefit from lateral decubitus positioning to prevent complications associated with prolonged supine or prone positions, ensuring optimal respiratory function and minimizing muscle strain.

Q133.

Answer: A.

Explanation: During anesthesia, padding the elbows helps prevent ulnar nerve compression, reducing the risk of nerve injury. Proper positioning techniques are crucial for patient safety and optimal outcomes during surgery.

Q134.

Answer B and D.

Explanation: Due to changes in lung mechanics, prone positioning may lead to reduced tidal volume and increased risk of hypercapnia. To prevent respiratory complications, monitoring these parameters is crucial.

Q135.

Answer A and C.

Explanation: Trendelenburg positioning is associated with increased venous return (preload) and may lead to an elevated heart rate. Understanding these physiological alterations is essential for effective anesthesia management.

Q136.

Answer: A and B.

Explanation: Due to pressure on the face and neck, prone positioning can lead to ocular compression and airway obstruction.

Q137.

Answer: A and B.

Explanation: Due to pressure on nerves and vessels in the pelvic region, the lithotomy position may cause nerve injury and impaired circulation to the lower extremities.

Q138.

Answer: B, C, D

Explanation: Arterial blood gas (ABG) assesses acid-base status, activated clotting time (ACT) evaluates coagulation, and liver function tests (LFTs) assess hepatic function, providing crucial data for perioperative management.

Q139.

Answer: B, D, E

Explanation: Activated clotting time (ACT), von Willebrand Factor Antigen, and Platelet Function Assay collectively assess primary and secondary hemostasis, crucial for safe perioperative management in patients with von Willebrand disease.

Q140.

Answers: C, E, F

Explanation: An elevated ST segment on the 12-lead ECG suggests myocardial ischemia. It is crucial for anesthesia providers to recognize this as it may influence perioperative management. Left bundle-branch block and ventricular tachycardia can also cause ST segment changes.

Q141.

Answers: C, D, E

Explanation: When interpreting a diagnostic exam an elevated hemidiaphragm, subsegmental atelectasis, and pleural effusion are preoperative chest X-ray is most concerning for the potential development of postoperative atelectasis. These should be carefully evaluated to optimize respiratory function and prevent complications.

Q142.

Answer: oropharyngeal

Explanation: To predict intubation difficulty, the Malampati classification assesses oropharyngeal structures. It aids in airway management decisions.

Q143.

Answer: thyroid notch

Explanation: The thyromental distance is measured from the thyroid notch to the chin. It helps assess airway patency and predicts potential difficulties in intubation.

Q144.

Answer: Jaw thrust

Explanation: By displacing the tongue forward without hyperextending the neck, the jaw thrust maneuver helps maintain airway patency.

Q145.

Answer: Endotracheal tube holder

Explanation: In airway procedures, the device commonly used to secure the endotracheal tube and prevent accidental extubation is called an endotracheal tube holder. It reduces the risk of displacement during patient care activities.

Q146.

Answer: C.

Explanation: During airway management, hypopharyngeal rupture may arise from improper positioning of the endotracheal tube cuff.

Q147.

Answer: A.

Explanation: To reduce the risk of complications associated with endotracheal intubation, in difficult airway situations, a Laryngeal mask airway (LMA) is favored during rapid sequence induction, especially when faced with challenging anatomy or limited visualization.

Q148.

Answer B.

Explanation: In the context of difficult airway management, the bougie airway device is specifically designed for use in patients with limited mouth opening.

Q149.

Answer A.

Explanation: In difficult airway situations, etomidate is the preferred induction agent, ensuring rapid onset and minimizing cardiovascular depression, making it suitable for compromised patients.

Q150.

Answer: A and B.

Explanation: To avoid complications and ensure effective regional anesthesia, administering an axillary nerve block requires awareness of the proximity of the brachial plexus and the location of the ulnar nerve.

Q151.

Answer: C and D.

Explanation: Avoiding inadvertent dural puncture is essential in lumbar epidural placement. To ensure accurate needle placement and prevent complications, knowledge of the ligamentum flavum and transverse process is critical.

Q152.

Answer A and D.

Explanation: Bradycardia can occur due to systemic absorption of the local anesthetic affecting the cardiovascular system, while local tissue necrosis may result from inadvertent intravascular injection.

Q153.

Answer A and C.

Explanation: In regional anesthesia, increased duration of action and enhanced nerve blockade are most likely associated with the use of epinephrine in local anesthetic solutions during infiltration.

Q154.

Answer: C, E, F.

Explanation: In the oral cavity, Tetracaine, benzocaine, and ropivacaine are frequently employed topically for mucosal anesthesia. Tetracaine provides rapid and potent local anesthesia, while benzocaine and ropivacaine offer alternative options with varying durations of action.

Q155.

Answer: C, D, F.

Explanation: During the neuraxial block, an unintentional vascular puncture may lead to hematoma formation, bradycardia, and infection. It highlights the importance of proper technique and anatomical knowledge.

Q156.

Answer: A, C, D.

Explanation: Hematoma formation, catheter dislodgement, and nerve injury are associated with continuous peripheral nerve block catheters. It can impact patient safety and recovery.

Q157.

Answer: A, D, F.

Explanation: Bupivacaine, ropivacaine, and articaine are commonly associated with a risk of systemic toxicity, causing initial CNS stimulation and subsequent depression. In various anesthesia practices, understanding the differences in local anesthetic profiles is crucial for safe administration.

Q158.

Answer: Epinephrine

Explanation: By reducing systemic absorption, combining local anesthetics with epinephrine vasoconstrictor prolongs the effect enhancing anesthesia duration, and minimizing bleeding at the injection site.

Q159.

Answer: Temporally near the ear

Explanation: To minimize the risk of globe penetration, the proper technique involves inserting the needle temporally near the ear, ensuring effective anesthesia for ophthalmic procedures.

Q160.

Answer: Sodium

Explanation: Local anesthetics exert their effects by blocking sodium channels, and inhibiting nerve impulse conduction. It leads to temporary anesthesia in the targeted area.

Q161.

Answer: Intralipid

Explanation: For local anesthetic systemic toxicity, Intralipid is used as a specific antidote. It works by creating lipid sinks, eliminating toxins, and improving cardiovascular stability.

Q162.

Answer A.

Explanation: In monitored anesthesia care (MAC), propofol is often chosen for light sedation due to its quick onset and short duration, allowing for easy titration and rapid recovery.

Q163.

Answer A and B.

Explanation: Chronic pain is influenced by psychological factors such as anxiety and depression, which can increase pain perception. Addressing these factors is important for comprehensive pain management.

Q164.

Answer B.

Explanation: In monitored anesthesia care, remifentanil is an appropriate choice for deep sedation because it provides effective analgesia and sedation without causing respiratory depression. Its short half-life allows precise control during the procedure.

Q165.

Answer: A.

Explanation: The high lipid solubility of propofol allows rapid onset and offset of anesthesia, making it ideal for total intravenous anesthesia. It facilitates induction and maintenance and distributes rapidly into the central nervous system.

Q166.

Answer: C.

Explanation: Remifentanil in total intravenous anesthesia is advantageous because it allows precise titration of analgesia without prolonged effects. Remifentanil is metabolized by nonspecific esterases, resulting in predictable effects and rapid elimination.

Q167.

Answer C and D.

Explanation: Pain modulation involves the release of neurotransmitters such as endorphins, which inhibit pain signals, and glutamate, which facilitates pain transmission.

Q168.

Answer A and C.

Explanation: Gabapentin is used to manage acute pain, particularly neuropathic pain, in perioperative settings. Morphine is a powerful opioid analgesic that is often used for postoperative pain relief.

Q169.

Answer A and C.

Explanation: Duloxetine, a serotonin-norepinephrine reuptake inhibitor (SNRI), and tramadol, an opioid analgesic, are commonly prescribed for chronic neuropathic pain because of their efficacy in modulating pain pathways and reducing pain perception.

Q170.

Answer: D, E, F.

Explanation: In the Enhanced Recovery After Surgery (ERAS) protocol, acetaminophen, gabapentin, and lidocaine are often included for their role in multimodal analgesia, promoting better recovery and reducing opioid use.

Q171.

Answer: A, E, F.

Explanation: Enhanced Recovery After Surgery (ERAS) protocols use multimodal analgesia and other techniques to reduce opioid use, expedite the return of bowel function, improve overall patient outcomes, and effectively manage postoperative pain.

Q172.

Answer B, D, F.

Explanation: Monitoring and prompt intervention are critical to maintaining patient safety, as hypotensive techniques may cause bradycardia, tachypnea, and increased intracranial pressure, which pose risks during anesthesia.

Q173.

Answer C, D, E.

Explanation: Nitroglycerin, sodium nitroprusside, and clevidipine agents are commonly used to induce controlled hypotension during hypotensive anesthesia. These agents help maintain optimal blood pressure levels during certain surgical procedures, thereby reducing the risk of bleeding.

Q174.

Answer: Deep tendon reflexes

Explanation: Early detection of magnesium toxicity is crucial, and monitoring deep tendon reflexes helps identify the initial signs, ensuring timely intervention.

Q175.

Answer: Pain pathways in the spinal cord

Explanation: Intrathecal narcotics modulate pain signals within the spinal cord, leading to altered pain perception without affecting proprioception or causing skeletal muscle weakness.

Q176.

Answer: D, E, F.

Explanation: The crucial infection control measures for anesthesia providers to prevent airborne transmission in the operating room are wearing N95 respirators to filter out airborne pathogens, utilizing face shields to protect mucous membranes, and donning hair covers to minimize contamination.

Q177.

Answer: B, E, F.

Explanation: Appropriate use of ultraviolet sanitizers involves consideration of factors such as the presence of laminar airflow, compatibility with electronic equipment, and distance from the UV source to ensure effective disinfection without compromising safety.

Q178.

Answer: B and C.

Explanation: For infection control in the anesthesia workplace, personal protective equipment and aseptic technique should be ensured during the procedure. These measures help reduce the risk of pathogen transmission and maintain a sterile environment, protecting both healthcare providers and patients.

Q179.

Answer A.

Explanation: High-flow oxygen increases the risk of fire. Minimizing its delivery and avoiding flammable substances are crucial to preventing intraoperative fires.

Q180.

Answer A.

Explanation: Selecting materials with flame-retardant properties is critical to intraoperative fire safety. This helps reduce the risk of fire in the operating room.

Q181.

Answer: D.

Explanation: Hepatobiliary surgery carries the risk of hepatic ischemia-reperfusion injury, making it critical to optimize perfusion and reduce ischemic time to prevent complications like liver failure.

Q182.

Answer: D.

Explanation: Aspiration pneumonitis should be closely monitored due to its potential impact on patient outcomes during anesthesia for gastrointestinal tract procedures.

Q183.

Answer: D.

Explanation: Hypoglycemia is of particular concern due to its potential impact on metabolic homeostasis during anesthesia for endocrine organ procedures. To prevent complications, close monitoring, and appropriate management are crucial.

Q184.

Answer: D.

Explanation: Acute tubular necrosis may result from intraoperative factors such as hypotension, hypovolemia, or nephrotoxic agents, which compromise renal function during and after surgery.

Q185.

Answer: D.

Explanation: Trendelenburg positioning can lead to uterine atony by increasing venous return and uterine blood flow, potentially causing postoperative hemorrhage in gynecologic surgeries.

Q186.

Answer: C.

Explanation: Pneumoperitoneum during laparoscopic procedures may cause hypercarbia because of carbon dioxide absorption which leads to respiratory acidosis and cardiovascular compromise if not managed appropriately.

Q187.

Answer: C.

Explanation: Impaired wound healing is of primary concern due to its potential impact on surgical outcomes, during anesthesia for extrathoracic plastics and reconstructive procedures.

Q188.

Answer: A.

Explanation: The facial nerve is at risk for injury due to its proximity to surgical sites, during head extracranial otolaryngological procedures such as facial surgeries.

Q189.

Answer: D.

Explanation: Invasive intracranial pressure monitoring allows direct pressure measurement within the cranial vault, which is important for detecting and managing intracranial hypertension during neurosurgical procedures.

Q190.

Answer: D.

Explanation: Intraoperative neurophysiologic monitoring is essential to detect cerebral perfusion changes and prevent cerebral ischemia as it includes techniques such as EEG, evoked potentials, and nerve stimulation.

Q191.

Answer: C.

Explanation: St. Thomas solution is commonly used to induce cardiac arrest during anesthesia for open cardiac procedures such as CABG.

Q192.

Answer: D.

Explanation: During TAVR/TAVI, preventing aortic regurgitation is the primary hemodynamic goal to optimize cardiac output and minimize myocardial injury.

Q193.

Answer: B.

Explanation: Monitoring for signs of pneumothorax is crucial to prevent device dislodgment and ensure proper lead placement during anesthesia for pacemaker implantation.

Q194.

Answer: C.

Explanation: During anesthesia for a patient with an intraarterial balloon pump, ensuring proper positioning of the arterial catheter is crucial to prevent malposition-related complications such as limb ischemia or arterial injury.

Q195.

Answer: D.

Explanation: Diaphragmatic surgery carries the risk of phrenic nerve injury due to its closeness to the surgical site which potentially leads to postoperative respiratory distress.

Q196.

Answer: C.

Explanation: Airway manipulation and potential trauma may lead to hypoxemia, requiring vigilant monitoring and intervention to maintain oxygenation.

Q197.

Answers: B and C.

Explanation: Esophageal surgery holds risks of esophageal perforation and subsequent mediastinitis which necessitates careful intraoperative monitoring and immediate recognition of potential complications.

Q198.

Answers: A and C.

Explanation: The nurse anesthetist should be vigilant for bronchopleural fistula and pneumothorax during anesthesia for lung surgery.

Q199.

Answers: A and C.

Explanation: Mediastinal surgery carries risks of tracheal compression due to mass effect and esophageal perforation from surgical manipulation, emphasizing the need for careful intraoperative monitoring and prompt intervention.

Q200.

Answers: A and B.

Explanation: Procedures involving the neck can lead to complications such as airway edema and vocal cord paralysis. To ensure optimal outcomes for the patient, careful monitoring and management are necessary.

Q201.

Answers: B and C.

Explanation: Neck lymph node biopsies can lead to bleeding because of the vascular structures and nerve injury due to proximity to vital nerves. This necessitates vigilant monitoring and prompt intervention to mitigate complications.

Q202.

Answers: A and B.

Explanation: Preventing hypotension ensures adequate perfusion to delicate structures, while monitoring recurrent laryngeal nerve integrity helps prevent nerve injury. These considerations are crucial for preserving vocal cord function during surgery.

Q203.

Answers: B and C.

Explanation: During delicate procedures, administering muscle relaxants ensures adequate surgical conditions while avoiding excessive head movement minimizes the risk of neural injury.

Q204.

Answers: B and C.

Explanation: Monitoring for compartment syndrome is crucial due to the risk of increased pressure in closed spaces. On the other hand, maintaining normothermia helps prevent perioperative complications and improves patient outcomes.

Q205.

Answers: B and C.

Explanation: During anal/rectal procedures, continuous monitoring of bowel motility helps prevent complications like postoperative ileus, while adequate pain control ensures patient comfort and facilitates early mobilization.

Q206.

Answers: B and D.

Explanation: During vascular surgery, the complexity of the lesion and anatomy often dictates whether open or endovascular procedures are suitable, while the surgeon's preference and experience play a significant role in selecting the approach.

Q207.

Answers: B and C.

Explanation: During extremity procedures, ensuring adequate perfusion through arterial cannulation is essential for managing occlusive disease, while monitoring peripheral pulses and administering regional anesthesia help maintain appropriate vascular access and perfusion.

Q208.

Answers: A and B.

Explanation: In the context of anesthesia for thromboembolic prevention, administering anticoagulant medications helps prevent clot formation, and vigilant monitoring for bleeding complications is crucial. Additionally, pneumatic compression devices and maintaining normothermia further reduce the risk of thromboembolism during anesthesia.

Q209.

Answers: A and B.

Explanation: In the surgical management of portal hypertension, selective portal vein embolization and transjugular intrahepatic portosystemic shunt (TIPS) are used to reduce portal pressure. Splenectomy and devascularization procedures are employed to address hypersplenism and variceal bleeding, respectively.

Q210.

Answers: A and D.

Explanation: During robotic/laparoscopic surgery, elevated intra-abdominal pressure during insufflation can impair venous return and lead to decreased cardiac output, while reducing intra-abdominal pressure post-operatively can improve cardiac function and reduce complications.

Q211.

Answers: A, C, F.

Explanation: The anatomical features of the airway in pediatric patients include a relatively larger and U-shaped epiglottis, a shorter and more flexible trachea, and a smaller tongue.

Q212.

Answers: A, B, D.

Explanation: Pediatric patients have a higher surface area-to-volume ratio, reduced subcutaneous fat for insulation, and immature thermoregulatory mechanisms. These factors make them more prone to hypothermia during anesthesia.

Q213.

Answers: B, C, E.

Explanation: Premature neonates often have immature thermoregulation, underdeveloped pulmonary surfactant production, and limited glycogen stores. These factors lead to an increased risk of hypoglycemia in these infants.

Q214.

Answers: D, E, F.

Explanation: Compered to term neonates, premature neonates have fewer alveoli, increased airway resistance, and a thinner and less complaint chest wall.

Q215.

Answers: A, D, F.

Explanation: Spina bifida, tracheoesophageal fistula, and cleft lip and palate are congenital abnormalities. They result from the failure of the neural tube, tracheoesophageal septum, and facial structures to close during embryonic development, respectively.

Q216.

Answers: B, C, E.

Explanation: In pediatrics, fentanyl, hydromorphone, and methadone are preferred due to their shorter duration of action and minimal accumulation compared to morphine, oxycodone, and codeine.

Q217.

Answers: C, D, F.

Explanation: Commonly used techniques for pediatric peripheral nerve blocks to provide regional anesthesia include brachial plexus block, fascia iliaca compartment block, and axillary nerve block.

Q218.

Answers: A, C, E.

Explanation: Aspiration, esophageal intubation, and hypoxemia are complications associated with pediatric airway management using a layered mask airway (LMA). These complications can occur due to inadequate ventilation or airway obstruction.

Q219.

Answers: A, C, D.

Explanation: During pregnancy, anatomical changes such as decreased gastric emptying, elevated diaphragm position, and reduced intra-abdominal pressure occur. These changes collectively increase the risk of aspiration during anesthesia.

Q220.

Answers: A, C, D.

Explanation: In tocolysis, pharmacological agents such as ritodrine, ephedrine, and ketorolac are commonly used to prevent preterm labor and fetal distress. These agents work by inhibiting uterine contractions or reducing inflammation.

Q221.

Answers: A, C, D.

Explanation: The preferred methods for labor analgesia in patients desiring mobility include continuous epidural analgesia, intermittent bolus epidural analgesia, and combined spinal-epidural analgesia. These procedures offer effective pain relief while allowing the laboring patients to move freely.

Q222.

Answers: A, B, D.

Explanation: When managing a high-risk parturient with a history of placenta accreta during cesarean delivery requires careful consideration. This includes ensuring blood product availability, implementing obstetric hemorrhage protocols, and conducting preoperative multidisciplinary discussions.

Q223.

Answers: A, B, D.

Explanation: Ensuring fetal well-being during Non-obstetric surgery in a parturient with placenta previa necessitates regional anesthesia to minimize bleeding risk, general anesthesia with rapid sequence induction, and continuous fetal heart rate monitoring.

Q224.

Answers: A, C, E.

Explanation: To improve maternal and fetal outcomes in suspected amniotic fluid embolism (AFE), prompt initiation of CPR, emergent cesarean delivery for fetal distress, and rapid institution of advanced airway management are essential interventions.

Q225.

Answers: A, E, F.

Explanation: Augmenting uterine contraction and controlling postpartum hemorrhage commonly involves the use of oxytocin, methylergonovine, and misoprostol pharmacologic agents.

Q226.

Answers: B, F, and E.

Explanation: Decreased renal function, reduced volume of distribution due to decreased lean body mass, and altered pharmacokinetics are often present in elderly patients, resulting in drug accumulation and prolonged effects.

Q227.

Answer: increased

Explanation: Careful titration and monitoring are required as they commonly experience increased sensitivity to opioids in geriatric patients to avoid adverse effects.

Q228.

Answer: dose or concentration

Explanation: To mitigate the risk of systemic toxicity and ensure effective anesthesia, geriatric patients often require lower doses or concentrations of local anesthetics during regional anesthesia.

Q229.

Answer: delirium

Explanation: Postoperative delirium frequently occurs in elderly patients, posing a risk factor for the development of postoperative cognitive dysfunction. Early recognition and management of delirium symptoms are crucial to minimize the impact of postoperative cognitive dysfunction.

Q230.

Answer: upper airway anatomy

Explanation: Upper airway anatomy changes due to obesity, such as fat deposition around the neck and pharynx, can lead to airway obstruction and difficulty with mask ventilation for patients.

Q231.

Answer: propofol

Explanation: Obesity can modify adipose tissue distribution and metabolism, thereby impacting the pharmacokinetics of lipophilic drugs like propofol. This alterations leads to changes in their volume of distribution.

Q232.

Answer: video laryngoscopy

Explanation: Due to its improved visualization of the airway structures, video laryngoscopy is favored in bariatric anesthesia, commonly aiding in difficult intubation situations in obese patients.

Q233.

Answer: obstructive sleep apnea (OSA)

Explanation: An elevated risk of airway obstruction and hypoventilation during anesthesia is frequently encountered in patients with obesity and comorbid OSA. It is crucial to recognize and address OSA for optimal perioperative management.

Q234.

Answer: opioid tolerance

Explanation: Opioid tolerance is frequently prevalent in patients on MAT, such as methadone or buprenorphine. It requires careful titration of opioids to prevent inadequate pain control or respiratory system.

Q235.

Answer: pharmacologic

Explanation: Changes in drug metabolism and increased sensitivity to anesthetics can occur due to acute intoxication, resulting in unpredictable responses and potential complications.

Q236.

Answer: analgesic

Explanation: Optimizing pain relief, minimizing opioid use, reducing the risk of addiction, and enhancing postoperative recovery are the primary goals of multimodal pain management.

Q237.

Answer: adverse events

Explanation: Careful monitoring and prompt intervention to mitigate complications is necessary for substance use disorder patients who are at increased risk for adverse events during anesthesia.

Q238.

Answer: immunosuppression

Explanation: The primary goals of anesthetic pharmacology in immune-compromised and oncology patients are to avoid complications and preserve immune function, thereby reducing the risk of immunosuppression.

Q239.

Answer: central line placement

Explanation: To minimize the risk of infections and associated complications, maintaining a strict aseptic technique during central line placement is vital in immune-compromised and oncology patients.

Q240.

Answer: hemodynamic status

Explanation: Close hemodynamic monitoring facilitates timely intervention to manage potential complications during anesthesia in immune-compromised and oncology patients.

Reward for the Readers

Scan QR Code Below to Claim the reward

Reward -1

Audio Book of Full-length practice test of NBCRNA Exam

240 Question in each practice test with answer explanation (MP3 Format)

Reward -2

200 Flash Cards (in Anki App format)

Made in the USA
Columbia, SC
14 February 2025